About the Author

William Long wrote this book after his experiences of helping his family care for his mum.
As well as being a published author William is a speaker on carer issues. He enjoys writing, reading, sports and travel. He is a keen runner and cyclist. He lives in Bishop's Stortford and is a manager in the public sector.

TO MUM AND DAD

THANK YOU FOR THE GREAT GIFT OF BEING
FINE PARENTS.

William Long

A GIFT FOR CARERS

- A PERSONAL GROWTH GUIDE FOR CARERS

- USE THE MINDSET SOLUTION TO INCREASE
YOUR HAPPINESS, HEALTH AND SUCCESS, WHILE
YOU CARE FOR SOMEONE YOU LOVE.

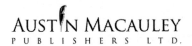
AUSTIN MACAULEY
PUBLISHERS LTD.

A CIP catalogue record for this title is available from the British Library.

ISBN 978 1 78455 230 5 (Paperback)
ISBN 978 1 78455 232 9 (Hardback)

www.austinmacauley.com

First Published (2015)
Austin Macauley Publishers Ltd.
25 Canada Square
Canary Wharf
London
E14 5LB

Printed and bound in Great Britain

Acknowledgments

There is not space here to thank all the people who provided me with the inspiration and knowledge necessary to write this book. I have truly stood on the shoulders of many giants in this writing process. These giants include Jim Rohn, Tony Robbins, Brian Tracy, Dennis Waitley, Stuart Goldsmith, Andy Shaw, Zig Ziglar, Bob Proctor, Brendon Burchard, Jack Canfield, Wayne Dyer and Eckhart Tolle. You have my undying respect and gratitude for your commitment to your craft, your teachings and your generosity of spirit.

As for the carers of the world, I salute you. It is our struggles that inspired me to write this book. I realise that the path of a carer can be a pretty dark one at times. It is my wish that this book helps to light up that path for you.

I must pay tribute to the publishers who have both shown faith in me and championed a worthy cause. Thanks for all your hard work and guidance that has allowed this book to happen.

To conclude I have three special thanks –

Firstly I want to thank my family for their support in looking after Mum all those years. This is also a legacy to your care and love.

Secondly I must thank my Mum for being the reason why this book was written. Thank you for showing me how to care.

Lastly I must thank Andy Harrington for instilling in me the belief that anything is possible.

INTRODUCTION

"It is in your moments of decision that your destiny is shaped" – Anthony Robbins.

My story

Have you ever had the feeling that life is like a bowl of cherries? Everything is easy, pleasurable and fun. Well this was my earlier life. Worry and fear were for other people only. I had a good job, great friends and a care free (some irony there) lifestyle. Looking back I realise that I took my good fortune for granted. I suppose that is just human nature.

Then one day I was around my mum's and she insisted, as always, in cooking me a nice roast dinner. As we were tidying up afterwards, I could not help but notice that her left arm was shaking. She told me that this had been going on a while and we agreed she would go to see her doctor about this. The doctor referred Mum onto a specialist. Little did I know, as I drove my mum to hospital that sunny September day, that both our lives were about to change forever.

I remember my mum's name being called out as we sat in the hospital waiting room. We duly entered the room marked Mr Stevens. There sat a distinguished looking man with half-rimmed spectacles balancing on the end of his nose. They added to his aura of intelligence and importance. He welcomed us in and then said that he had the results of the tests back. At this point he paused, took off his glasses, put his hands together and looked up to the ceiling as if he was searching for the right words. He then turned his gaze on my mum and said something like: "Mrs Long, I'm afraid I have some bad news for you. The results show that you have the early signs of Parkinson's disease." I cannot recall what he said after that as I was reeling from the shock of this information.

As we drove back home we were both silent, being lost in our own thoughts. I remember squeezing her hand as I saw tears welling up in her eyes. I was lost for words of comfort at that point and that short drive felt like an eternity.

As the years passed Mum's condition worsened. Gradually I found myself, more and more, helping her with her daily tasks. Although this made me closer to Mum it came at a price. Slowly I started to feel the effects of exhaustion and was feeling mentally down on an increasing basis. My social life became almost non-existent and friends stopped inviting me to social events. I felt increasingly isolated from them. I realise now that I was probably suffering from low level depression. My solution? I simply self-medicated with alcohol most nights. We all find ways to cope although mine was not the best, I think you will agree. At times I felt total despair. I did not realise there were organisations like Carers UK who were waiting to help me. I was probably too proud and stubborn to ask for help anyway.

After ten years of caring for Mum it became obvious that she needed a higher level of care. The carers that the local authority provided were kind and did their best.

They were just ordinary people doing a difficult job on minimum wages. My mum had also developed a related dementia condition. After much persuasion and after several stays in hospital my mum consented to go into a care home.

In the next few months my health was boosted as I regained my life. There was still a nagging sense of guilt over whether I could have done more. However I knew that she was in the best place and the home would make her last few years comfortable ones.

Why did I write this book?

They even have a name for it: Caregiver Syndrome. This is the term given to the long term effects of caring for someone. The psychological and physical effects can indeed be devastating over a period of time. Often when we care for someone we put our own needs on hold. Depression, exhaustion and anxiety can creep up on us as a result.

I have always enjoyed reading. On one visit to the library (an old fashioned concept I know) I looked at all the books written for carers. I noticed that there were many books on how to care for people with many different and varied conditions. These are all great books, I am sure and well worth reading. However I could not find a book that focused solely on the wellbeing of the carer. Through my reading I had developed a passion for self-development. These books gave me hope and strength to carry on. They were also healthier than alcohol. I particularly was inspired by the stories of ordinary people who had overcome great challenges and had gone on to build great lives. I realised that if these books had helped me then they could help others.

I had discovered a "gap in the market" if you like. My intention for you is to read this book and take action. It is my job in these pages, to change the whole way you view your current situation. Indeed, to see your situation as a gift. A gift that will inspire you to improve your happiness, your health and very possibly your wealth. It is said that the last thing that was drawn out of Pandora's Box was hope. I think we could all do with a little more hope.

In this book I will cover seven crucial areas for your personal growth. I will also give you action steps to reinforce your knowledge. These steps will be quick, cost little or no money and are designed to be fun. This is a practical book written by an ordinary guy. The only knowledge that will help you is applied knowledge. Indeed, I believe that you only really know something if you apply it.

This is certainly not an academic text book. It is full of examples and stories that you will find engaging and inspiring. I have tried to explain complex subjects, such as psychology, in simple day to day language. This will be a fascinating journey of self-discovery. At times it might unmask some "little demons." Just keep going and remember you are venturing where most people fear to tread. You will know and like yourself much better. You will tap into your inner genius. You will discover how incredible you are and all those around you. You will undergo change. You will feel uncomfortable at times. This is good as you are expanding your comfort zone. Many treasures, both large and small await you. The more you put into this, the more you will get out of yourself. Your energy and enthusiasm will increase as you realise that you are taking control of your thoughts and life. Enjoy.

Why Now?

It is estimated that 70% of carers (care givers in the U.S.) suffer from depression. The aim of this book is primarily to enable the reader to take a proactive approach to ensure their happiness. Happiness is a skill and all skills can be learnt. We will discover what truly makes us happy. It is definitely not what society and the media would have us believe.

When I researched this problem I was astonished at the wider problems in society. According to the charity MIND, 3 out of 4 people will suffer from some form of mental illness in their lifetime. All addiction rates have increased over the last few decades. These include drugs, alcohol, food and gambling. The biggest killer of men under the age of 35 is suicide. I assumed it was motorbikes or alcohol. Self-harming has almost reached epidemic proportions in teenagers. In a recent study of young people it emerged that the majority of those taking part feared that they would have a worse life than their parents. Ok, I will stop there as this is enough to realise that there is a serious lack of happiness in people.

With state funding being cut back throughout the western world, I believe that we all need to take control of our emotional and physical wellbeing. We cannot abdicate this responsibility to anyone else. It is too important to leave to chance.

Happiness versus pleasure

It is important that we first define what happiness is. Happiness is a level of contentment. Unlike pleasure it is a feeling of wellbeing, gratitude and connection. It is a connection to our naturally happy self. Pleasure can give us a quick hit of happiness but we must not confuse the two. We get pleasure from a good meal. We get happiness from a great relationship. There is nothing wrong with pleasure but we again must not confuse the two. Pleasures, such as over eating or drinking are fun in the moment. They do not lead to lasting happiness.

My solution

This book covers my MINDSET solution to the above problems. It covers seven key areas that we can strengthen. These are the seven secrets to lasting, sustainable health and happiness. If you work on any one of these areas you should see results. The more areas you work on the better and the more permanent will be your progress. You cannot rush change so just read when you can and apply the techniques that feel right. The important thing is to keep making steady progress. Remember the tortoise and the hare. This is not a race against anyone.

Back to my story

If you had been with me on 21st March 2012 you would have been in my mum's room in a nursing home in a village in Essex, England. You would have seen my mum in the last days of her life and asleep. At the foot of the bed my toddler niece was playing and blissfully unaware of the situation. Opposite me sat my tearful sister.

I am sure you have experienced a moment like this when you are trying to find a positive meaning. I was lost in my own thoughts at this point – was this the end or a new beginning? Should I feel relief or just heartbroken? Suddenly I became aware that my mum had opened her eyes and seemed to be staring directly at me. I had been deep in my thoughts and this gave me a start. In an instant I felt a shiver run down my spine as she seemed to be saying "You're next son so start living!"

Many, many years ago, in a faraway land, there lived an old farmer. One day he was out walking in a field when he spotted a baby bird that had fallen from its nest. Carefully the old man picked up the bird and took it home. Over the next few months the old farmer reared the bird in a small bamboo cage he kept in his garden. It soon grew up with beautiful feathers and was by now far too big for the cage.

Every day the bird begged the farmer to release it so that the bird could stretch its wings. The old man always refused for fear that the bird, now his only companion, would escape. One morning the farmer went into his garden and found the bird motionless, apparently dead at the bottom of the cage. The farmer opened the cage door in despair. At that moment the bird flew straight out of the cage and landed on a tree branch nearby.

The farmer angrily shouted at the bird; "Why did you trick me when I have cared for you all this time?" The bird simply looked down on him and said; "In order to set myself free, I realised I would have to die before I died." That is what I had done in my mum's room that spring day. I had glimpsed my own mortality for the first time. I realised that it was now my duty to live my life fully. And with that thought I stood up and walked over to my mum. I leant over, kissed her on the forehead and whispered "I love you" for the first and only time in my life. I then left the room. My mum passed away 3 days later.

A turning point

Eighteen months later I was seated in the main auditorium at the Ed-excel centre in Docklands, London. The event was a personal development seminar. If again you had been seated with me you would have witnessed an event that changed my life and might well have changed yours. At around midday a speaker took to the stage who I found so inspiring that I decided I wanted more than anything to be able to influence and inspire people like he could. The speaker's name was Andy Harrington and I remember he said something like; "Why have you spent your whole life trying to fit in when you were born to stand out?" That day I promised myself that I would find a way to contribute. It is my sincere wish that this book contributes positively to your future.

Universal laws

Before we start to get into more detail, I want to cover some fundamental laws which affect us all.

The first law is the law of cause and effect. This has been described as the iron law of the universe so it is worth discussing. The law simply states that for any effect (results, outcomes) there are causes (reasons). This is the biblical law of sowing and reaping. Another way of putting this is that success and failure both leave clues. This law is so important because we must now accept that we are responsible for our results in life. It means we have the power to change our lives.

The second law is the law of attraction. Quantum physics has proved that everything in the universe is energy. This means that our thoughts are energy. If we think negatively we create negative energy which attracts more negative energy. Conversely if we think positive thoughts we attract positive energy into our lives. Put simply, positive people lead positive lives and negative people .... Well you get the idea. The book *The Secret* covers this well. If you want scientific proof type in "The double slit experiment" into YouTube. I would warn you that quantum physics is very weird so you have to just go with it.

The third important law is the law of correspondence. This law states that your outer world is a projection of your inner world. Karl Jung, the famous psychologist stated that "perception is projection." Simply put, how we think about all areas of our life determines our results, attitudes and beliefs we project into the world. Our thoughts create our life and reality. If we change our thinking we change our lives.

The benefits of this book

After reading this book you will gain the following:-

- Higher levels of self-esteem
- An improvement in your physical health
- A greater understanding of yourself and others
- A powerful mind-set

- A more optimistic outlook
- The ability to handle change
- The confidence just to be yourself
- Greater focus and a sense of direction
- A general feeling of contentment and wellbeing.

OK, let's get started with the M in MINDSET which stands for…

CHAPTER ONE

MENTORS

"If I have seen further it is by standing on the shoulders of giants" – Sir Isaac Newton.

The year was 1908 and a young reporter was tasked with interviewing Andrew Carnegie who at the time was the world's richest man and America's first great industrialist. Carnegie was so impressed with the young reporter that he set him a challenge: Go and interview the most successful people and discover their secrets.

The young reporter gladly took on the challenge and over the next twenty years interviewed over twenty-five thousand of the wealthiest people in America. Eventually in 1937 this reporter named Napoleon Hill published *Think and Grow Rich*. This book has sold over twenty million copies and is still regarded as a classic. Hill had realised all those years before that he had found a great mentor, followed his advice and achieved international acclaim in the process.

It is said that Sir Richard Branson has five mentors at any one time. After I read that it figures that we need to take this subject seriously. The speaker and author M.R.

Kopmeyer wrote a large work where he listed one thousand success secrets he had discovered in his years of study. This work was vast and contained four volumes. He was once asked by a reporter what was the number one secret that if applied would help make someone successful. The reporter figured that most people don't want to read through four volumes but just want the number one secret. Mr Kopmeyer did not hesitate when he gave this answer. It was simply to... learn from the experts.

This is the greatest shortcut to getting any result you desire. We must find someone who has what we want and learn from them. Fortunately for us there are examples of success all around us. Many have written books that can light our way. Life is too short to figure stuff out for ourselves. We can save ourselves a lot of time, money and effort by copying someone else's strategies. Let's not get too obsessed with inventing our own wheel when there are plenty of great ones out there to copy.

We have had mentors all our lives and the first and most important were our parents. You have probably heard the old saying: 'The apple doesn't fall far from the tree'. As young children we looked at our parents as some sort of gods and believed anything they said. Indeed, without mentors we would not be able to walk. As a toddler we saw the adults walking around us and we decided that is what we wanted and of course we did not stop until we achieved this. (We will cover goal setting later.) Then as we grew up our school teachers became our role-models. We still remember with fondness the teachers we liked and conversely the ones we hated.

You may have heard that we become the average of the five or six adults that we most associate with in terms of income, health, and lifestyle choices etc. We fuss and worry about who our children associate with but forget that, we as adults, become whom we associate with.

Fleas in a jar

In a famous experiment scientists took some fleas and placed them in a glass jar with a clear glass top. The fleas of course tried to jump out of the jar and duly kept hitting the top. Eventually the scientists could remove the top and the fleas could not jump out of the jar. The scientists concluded that the fleas had conditioned their nervous systems that they could only jump to the top of the jar. Then they added some new fleas into the jar and left the top off. Surprisingly the new fleas did not jump out and stayed with the old fleas. Moral of this experiment: We will only jump as high as our associates.

Crabs in a box

If a fisherman catches a crab they place it in a box and put a lid on the box or else the crab will crawl out. However, once several crabs have been caught the fishermen can leave the lid off safe in the knowledge that any crab who attempts to leave the box will be pulled back by the other crabs. Similarly we are often held back by the disapproval of others. Please remember that if anyone tells you that you can't do something then what they are saying is that they don't think they can. Unfortunately we have all listened to these people and put our dreams on hold. Moral here: avoid crabs in a box or else they will pull you down!

If we go back to the subject of confidence and look it up in a dictionary we discover that it comes from the Latin verb fidere which means to trust. The word faith also stems from this root. If we have self-confidence it stands to reason that we trust ourselves. The areas we lack confidence in we can be sure we do not trust ourselves to perform well in. The reason we should always search for mentors is that we can trust that their company, experience and advice will be sound and beneficial. We must also have faith that we can confide in them which again is a form of trust.

Where are the mentors?

I read a statistic that only 1% of people at age 65 are worth one million US dollars or more. (I am talking in the western world here – the figures for the rest of the world are too depressing to print). What this means is that success is rare. Money is only one barometer of success but take any area (e.g. health) and we find few people are where they want to be.

All the success books I have read emphasise the importance of getting around the right people. My problem, which I suspect is common, was that I was surrounded by the 99%. Don't get me wrong, most of my friends and associates were good people and I felt comfortable around them. The problem was that I needed to find people who would hold me to a higher standard – but where?

Books and Autobiographies

The easiest place to look is reading the stories of other people. Most interesting to me were the stories of people who have overcome great difficulties to make a success of their lives. I found these stories inspiring and a great help in building my confidence in this belief: If you persist long enough you will succeed. Nothing, of course, builds confidence like success. One book I would highly recommend is *Man's Search for Meaning* by Viktor Frankl.

It was the 1930s and Frankl was a psychiatrist and university professor based in Germany. As an Austrian Jew in Hitler's Germany, he found himself imprisoned in a concentration camp. The only thing that kept him alive was his fascination with human behaviour. In the most extreme conditions imaginable he saw how some inmates gave up and died whilst others did whatever it took to survive this nightmare. He realised that he must survive so that he could tell his story to the world. Frankl and the other survivors had found a meaning amongst the horror which was to make sure this tragedy did not happen again. After the war Frankl wrote his great book and went on to become a world famous psychotherapist and invented the treatment called 'logotherapy'. I believe Frankl taught us that there is no inherent meaning in any situation, however bad, but the one we choose. Indeed, he is famous for saying that between stimulus (the event) and response (our reaction), we always have the freedom of choice. Can you see how that thought might help us?

Audio Learning

Researchers have known since the 1970s that people have different learning styles. If you don't want to read then listening to mentors is a great way to learn from them. The advantage of course is that you can be doing your chores and listening at the same time. I often listen to people such as Tony Robbins, Brian Tracy, Jim Rohn and others whilst I drive. This is also a great way to turn dead time into learning time. More importantly I find their enthusiasm and positive outlook contagious. When we listen to something positive it has an emotional effect. This increases our happiness and energy levels.

The Internet

Probably the best and cheapest place to track down experts is through internet searches. At the cost of giving away your email you can get some great content on the subjects that interest you. Within five years at least 70% of downloads will be in video format. Most people are catching on so a great source for this is of course YouTube. You can find and watch every expert on the planet there. This is another great use of your time. You are learning and ensuring that you stay in a positive state of mind at the same time.

Webinars and Seminars

The advantage of webinars are that you don't even have to leave your house to hear your expert's words of wisdom. If you miss them they are also usually recorded so you can listen at your convenience.

Seminars are a great place not only to meet experts in person but also to network with like-minded people. A few months back I was chatting to a guy sitting next to me who proudly told me he was having his book published. I thought to myself that if he could then why not me? It is strange how a chance meeting with a stranger can have such an influence on someone. Seminars give you the chance to immerse yourself in a subject for a day or more and you can ask questions. You get to mix with fleas that are jumping out of the jar.

Coaching

For those with deeper pockets one to one coaching is a great way to learn and get solutions and mentoring tailored to your unique circumstances. It can be very intense so choose someone you want to spend time with. A coach will also hold you accountable, offer support and should speed up your progress dramatically. Just remember that a coach is not your friend. They are your coach. Their job is to push you out of your comfort zone. You are paying them to get results.

Excuses

Obviously our mind-set affects the amount of action we will take. The attitude we have in factors outside ourselves greatly matter here. Our confidence in other people will decide what actions we will take such as delegating tasks. A big factor in our confidence is the economy. Economists study consumer and business confidence as these areas greatly affect our spending habits and our attitudes to risk taking. If all around us are screaming recession then we all tighten our belts and guess what happens? Then the press announces the recession is over and we all get out our credit cards. It is said that all financial markets are driven by greed and fear which is just another measure of confidence.

The point here is that we must be aware of what is happening around us but let's not use this as an excuse for non-action. Excuses are often lies we tell ourselves. It is a little known fact that during the great depression of the 1930s, America produced more millionaires than at any time in its history. I assume those folk who got rich were not listening to the media!

The Colonel

Colonel Harland Saunders was a chicken restaurant owner in Corbin, Kentucky, who went bust when they put a freeway over his little chicken shop. At the age of sixty-six he found himself dead broke and on welfare. In spite of all this, he asked himself one day: "What do I have that could help me out of this mess?" He realised he had a great chicken recipe so he spent two years travelling around America trying to convince businesses to partner him. After countless rejections and setbacks he decided to franchise his idea and KFC was born. By the time he was seventy-five Colonel Saunders was one of the richest men in the world. Whatever our excuse is, someone has overcome it.

Tony Robbins tells the story of how he interviewed two brothers. One brother was in prison on death row and asked him to explain his situation. He told Tony that his father was an alcoholic and that he had no choice in life but to end up as he did. He then interviewed the other brother who was enormously successful as a lawyer and businessman. Again Tony asked him to explain his situation and he stated that his father was an alcoholic and so he had to end up being successful. This is further proof that we can all let our difficulties inspire us or beat us. This is not easy but we now know it is possible.

Warning or example?

The late Jim Rohn used to say that our lives will serve as either a warning or an example to others. Luckily there are plenty of "ordinary people" we can model. As I write this I have just read an article of a group of limbless ex-soldiers who are skiing across the South Pole for charity. As I thought about this I realised that if they had returned home uninjured they would probably spend their time watching soap operas and moaning about the weather. (The weather is an obsession if you are British). Now obviously these guys have had a lot of counselling but they have somehow taken something bad happening (losing your legs we can agree would spoil most people's day) and have turned this into almost a gift to help the world. In ancient times alchemists used to attempt to turn dirt into gold and that is exactly what these young men and women have done.

NLP

The science of Neuro-Linguistic Programming (NLP) is a great tool to help explain human behaviour. One thing this science does is to teach us to model excellence. A good question we can ask someone who is confident in performing a certain task is: "How do you do that?" Most people like to share their advice so we must never miss a chance to learn from others. Another question is: "How would I act if I were confident at this task?" No doubt our voice would be steady and carry conviction. Our breathing would be full and our head and body upright. Our gestures would clearly reflect this. Getting a mental picture of yourself performing great things is very useful. There are many good books on this subject if this interests you.

Action points:

- What famous people past and present do you admire?
- Read their autobiographies and books.
- Research the internet for experts in your areas of interest. Download their material, listen to their videos and take notes.
- Ask someone you know and would like to model: "How do you do that?" Once they have got over the shock they will be happy to tell you.
- Imagine how you would talk, stand, walk and talk if you were really confident in any situation.
- Remind yourself that you are a role-model to many people so allow yourself to feel good about that.

In the next chapter we move onto a vital component of our happiness. The I in Mind-set stands for....

CHAPTER 2

INTEGRITY

"The cave you fear to enter holds the treasure you seek." – Joseph Campbell

All confident, happy, successful people have integrity. The word comes from *integer* which is Latin for whole or complete. Barbara Killinger offers an alternative definition: "Integrity is a personal choice, an uncompromising and predictably consistent commitment to honour moral, ethical, spiritual and artistic values and principles." In this chapter we are going to study, not just our moral integrity, but how we can unite mind, body and spirit to enhance our whole experience of life. This chapter offers a holistic approach which strengthens these three essential areas.

Let's explore these three elements further.

Values

Integrity is being congruent in our thoughts and actions. In other words we must live in harmony with our values. If you think about the people you most admire I bet that one of their characteristics is a strong sense of values. So where do our values come from? Our parents installed our first values into us from a young age and this continued as we became aware of our environment, our family and as we attended school. Psychologists state that most of our values are firmly in place by the age of ten. In view of this now might be a great time to review our values to make sure they are taking us where we want to go. Out of date values are like using an out of date road map: a large element of luck is needed to arrive at our chosen destination.

So how do we review our values? The writer Brian Tracy has a useful idea here. He suggests that you imagine that the eulogy is being read out at your funeral. What would you want the speaker to say about you? What values, attitudes, beliefs and characteristics would you like to have described you? What did you stand for? What did you fight for? What was your influence on others?

Going back to famous people we can often guess their values by their actions.

A young western reporter once followed Mother Teresa around for several days as this old nun tended to the poor, sick and dying in the slums of Calcutta, India. At the end of what had been a traumatic experience for the reporter, she interviewed her subject. She asked the old nun how she could appear to be so happy and at peace when constantly surrounded by the most severe poverty imaginable. Mother Teresa simply told her: "In each person I see, I see the face of Christ in one of his more distressing guises." That gives us a great insight into her character. Did you think that belief served her well in caring for others? No prizes for guessing that one of her top values was compassion and kindness.

Nelson Mandela was once asked what it was like to have suffered in prison for twenty-seven years. He replied that he had not suffered in all those years, but had spent the time preparing to lead and unite his country. Of course history tells us this is what he did. I am sure forgiveness was an important value to him.

International icon Oprah Winfrey was brought up in poverty and was the victim of appalling sexual abuse as a young girl. She has said, though, that she has come to terms with this and realised that her experiences have made her the woman she is today. Oprah continues to inspire millions of people around the world. One of her main values, I am sure, is contribution.

My countryman, Winston Churchill, was often a lone voice in the British Parliament opposing appeasement with Hitler. The British people listened to him when he insisted we fight for our freedom and a nation fought back against evil. Churchill's great value? Freedom.

I said at the introduction that this book was practical in its nature. I am going to ask you to think about and list your values. Very few people have thought much about this, let alone written them down. These are deep questions and this will take some thought. As someone once said, I am not here to sell easy. It took me a while to come up with my list but it felt great to have answered the questions above. Just take your time and give it some thought. There is no rush so just go for a walk or play your favourite music. There are no right or wrong answers here and there is no need to send your values in for marking. Just relax and try to list your values in some sort of order. Just write what feels right.

For thousands of years people have turned to philosophy and religion as guidance in this area. Christianity gives us the Ten Commandments and there is a treasure trove of advice in all these teachings. Strong values give us a great feeling of being grounded and this leads to greater self-esteem and happiness.

MY TOP TEN VALUES

GOD.
PEACE OF MIND.
HEALTH.
FAMILY.
LOVE AND KINDNESS.
HONESTY.
CONTRIBUTION.
FREEDOM.
GRATITUDE.
AWARENESS AND LEARNING.

OK how did I do? I have just limited myself to ten values here but obviously we have a multitude of values and sub-values. I could have included wealth and lifestyle, as these have a big impact on our happiness and wellbeing, but I think the above is a good start. There are, to repeat, no right or wrong answers but the great advantage of doing this is the mental clarity it gives you. Actually doing this exercise and the process of writing your values down will drive them deeper into your subconscious mind. Where your conscious mind responds to logic your subconscious mind responds to emotion.

Our subconscious mind is many times more powerful and we can access it by adding strong emotions to our values. Take some time to actually feel your values resonating inside your body. I find it easier if I close my eyes and imagine what it feels like to be loved and give love. If we can link strong positive emotions to our values they become like a powerful moral compass that will guide us through life's inevitable ups and downs.

Value conditions

Another area we must explore is the conditions and standards we place on ourselves to experience and therefore fully enjoy our values.

For example if someone's criteria for health is they must train five times a week down the gym, only eat fresh food and meditate three hours a day, the chances are that they will suffer disappointment sooner or later. Whilst it is good to have high standards, this person may find that if they relax these strict conditions they may enjoy life and their health more.

If we are to become obsessed with anything it should be to lead a balanced life. With demands that we and others place on ourselves we need to cut ourselves some slack otherwise we experience stress and overwhelm.

Be an underachiever

Success is often doing the simple things well. I used to be a gym fanatic who would train flat out two hours at a time four times a week. As I got older I realised this was just leaving me exhausted, irritable and was negatively impacting other areas of my life. After hearing this idea of underachieving I now just go to the gym and tell myself I will just train for thirty minutes. This has had several benefits: I enjoy exercising a lot more. I don't make excuses to myself such as I am too tired. I train more often. I feel a lot healthier which was the point of going in the first place!

I have applied this idea of little but often to all areas of my life and I find that I experience less stress and I get more done which of course increases my happiness. Progress equals happiness and we can get a lot of joy in making small steps towards our desires. Another reason I like this idea, is that I don't have to waste time motivating myself to do what needs to be done as I now enjoy these tasks more. We all know that the most powerful human driver is our need to move toward pleasure and away from pain. I have not used the F word yet but the more fun we can associate with our activities and values the better.

Try this idea yourself – the results might surprise you.

MY Ten Values and Conditions

GOD. – Every time I look in awe at nature I am close to God.

PEACE OF MIND – Every time I feel a sense of calmness.

HEALTH. – Every time I eat something healthy, exercise, meditate or rest.

FAMILY. – Every time I share experiences or spend time with them.

LOVE AND KINDNESS. – Every time I smile, give support or am nice to anyone.

HONESTY. – Every time I consider that my actions are moral.

CONTRIBUTION. – Every time I help anyone.

FREEDOM. – Every time I realise I have the freedom to choose.

GRATITUDE. – Every time I count my blessings.

AWARENESS AND LEARNING. – Every time I learn something.

Decisions, Decisions

Another benefit of clearly stating your values and value conditions is that it enables us to make faster decisions. Being decisive is a great attribute and greatly enhances our confidence and lives. Nothing is worse than being indecisive and I always get a feeling of relief when I make a firm decision. All confident, successful people make decisions quickly and change their decisions slowly. The mental clarity that values give us can be priceless.

An example of this would be a woman who was offered a new job at a much higher salary. Upon reflection she realised that this job would impact negatively her top values of family and health. Because she valued these areas more than money she decided to turn the job down.

The word decision comes from the Latin verb *decisio*, meaning to cut away. In making firm decisions we are therefore directing and controlling the focus, meaning and direction of our life.

Shifting Values

A challenge that faces many young people today is that they are unclear as to what their values should be. In today's society many youngsters are brought up in broken homes. The parents are doing the best they can in a difficult situation but it is inevitable that the philosophies of the two households are different as there would not have been a break up in the first place. This is further compounded by values taught in school, television and the social media culture we now live in. My advice here would be to make sure there is general agreement and compromise amongst all parties as to how the children will be raised. There are many good books on parenting that cover these problems.

BODY

The Japanese sportswear company ASICS take their name from the Latin phrase *Anima Sana In Corpore Sano* which comes from the writing of the Greek philosopher Thales. It translates as 'a healthy mind in a healthy body'. It seems that the ancient Greeks understood that the mind and body are intimately linked. Sadly the school system teaches us little about the importance of nutrition and as a society we are getting sicker. Even our medical system seems to focus on the effects (illness and disease) and not the causes, which is often our poor lifestyle choices. Our health simply plays a major part in our enjoyment of life.

Occam's razor

In the 13th century a philosopher by the name of William of Ockham put forward a principle which is now known as Occam's razor. What his principle stated is that, in problem solving, the simplest solution is often the best and that we should "shave" away more complex solutions – hence the word razor. Many great scientists have apparently used this principle throughout the centuries, in their work, including Einstein.

After a lifetime of thinking, Einstein simplified his entire scientific theories into one equation: $E=MC^2$. The conclusion here is that simplicity really can be genius.

OK so you are probably asking what the hell this has to do with our health. The point here is that in our modern society we are looking for ever more elaborate and complex solutions to achieve good health. I would argue that our natural state is good health and it is ours to claim back. Studies have shown that our grandparents were as a whole much slimmer and healthier than us without the need for gyms, fad diets and pills. They had a simple solution to health that worked. They went to bed early, got up early, ate healthy food and led active lives.

I strongly believe that success is about doing the little things well so let's look at what we can do to improve this critical area of our health.

Water

If we think about it our bodies are made up of over 70% water and our brains 80%. Unfortunately we forget this most basic need and spend our days drinking sugary drinks, tea and coffee, which often dehydrate us more. The simple message here is that you cannot drink enough water. Our bodies need water for every chemical reaction in the body so we cannot burn fat, and hence lose weight, if we are not properly hydrated. Most headaches (especially hangovers) are caused by dehydration and so are often those dips in energy during the day.

Try and start each day with at least one glass of water each day and continue sipping away. Do this and your skin will look better – that is why all models do this. Water flushes away excess salt and sugar so it lowers our blood pressure and helps us keep slim. There is magic in water and it's free.

Breathing

Every second of our lives we need oxygen. The human body was designed for movement and, because we are sedentary for a lot of our lives, we have forgotten to breathe properly. If we exercise we automatically breathe deeply which is one of the benefits of course. Ideally we should breathe in from our stomachs and not from our chests. A good breathing exercise is to sit or stand and breathe in by pulling in the stomach for a count of ten and breathing out by relaxing the stomach to another count of ten. You can do this five times whilst watching the TV or working at your computer and no one will notice. I read a study recently that said that people who sang in choirs enjoy better than average health and live longer lives. The study concluded that this is in part due to the excellent breathing work out singing provides, as well as the enjoyment and camaraderie. Breathing well reduces our stress levels. It is common for people to reach for a cigarette when under pressure. It is of course the act of breathing which calms them down and not the nicotine, which is a powerful stimulant – the placebo effect in action!

Exercise

Doctors tell us that if we were to go for a brisk twenty minute walk every day that would be enough to ensure ideal health and fitness. Indeed, I saw a programme on obesity last year which stated that the difference between being overweight and your ideal weight is as little as two thousand footsteps a day.

For some reason I used to avoid all exercise unless I was in the gym – crazy or what? What I mean is that we can keep in shape by always taking the stairs instead of the lift (unless you work in a skyscraper) and by simply cycling or walking whenever we can. It took me a while to realise that if I parked at the far side of the parking lot I would save myself hours of my life waiting for a space by the front door, and I got extra exercise in the meantime.

One critical distinction we have to make is the difference between health and fitness. The two are of course linked but not mutually exclusive. Health is the optimum working of all the body's systems i.e. heart, liver etc. Fitness is the body's ability to repeatedly perform an action i.e. running, press-ups etc. Ideally then we want to find an exercise plan that enhances both our fitness and health. As I have mentioned I have had to adapt my regime as I have got older to ensure some balance.

There are three main types of exercise we should consider. The first is cardio vascular. This is the most important and involves any stamina based activity such as running, rowing, walking, swimming, cycling etc. This exercise ensures that our heart and lungs are strong and gives us the endurance to enjoy life.

The second type are strength exercises. This often involves lifting weights. This area also covers resistance exercises such as push ups. A lot of women are scared of doing weights because they think they will bulk up. Research has shown that our metabolic rate is higher when we lift weights than when we do a cardiovascular workout. This is why we breathe so much after a single repetition of weights. So lifting light weights is actually a great way to burn fat. If you do not want to go to the gym then digging in the garden will have similar effects. Having a strong body not only gives us better posture but strength exercises strengthen our bones.

The third type are flexibility exercises. This includes all stretching and manipulation of the joints. Yoga, Pilates and Tai-chi are great for keeping the body supple and giving us a good range of movement.

The most important thing about all exercise is that, whilst giving us the desired results, it should be fun and not damage us. There are many books on this subject and please consult your doctor if you have any health concerns.

Healthy Eating

I have deliberately avoided the word diet here as all diets are doomed to fail. The first three letters of the dreaded word spell die, which I think I would rather do than diet. Why would anyone want to starve themselves so that they condition their bodies to go into emergency mode? This means they are now super-efficient at storing fat. When the inevitable happens and they cave in to temptation they are now in a great position to become fatter than when they started. This is how a person's weight yo-yos for years and is totally insane. As humans we are designed to eat and enjoy our food. The problem is that our bodies' genetics have not changed since we lived in caves and so we are not exactly prepared for the modern diet of processed foods.

As a society where obesity rates are alarming, even in our children, we really need to go back to basics here. As someone who loves his food, I realise that I need to focus more on what I eat and not on how much I eat. For change to be lasting and to enjoy a lifetime of good health (which is our natural state) we need to focus on eating lots of healthy food with the occasional treat thrown in. This takes discipline at first but if we remember that "nothing tastes as good as being slim feels" we can all, over time, claim the right to a healthy, happy life.

It all comes down to picking up new healthier habits and letting go of the old unhealthy ones, as they no longer serve us. I will therefore share with you what has worked for me. Everyone is different so I encourage you to research and experiment as to which foods work best for you. Hippocrates, the father of modern medicine, once said: "Let food be your medicine, let medicine be your food." Wise words indeed.

<u>Go Green</u>

It seems that our grandparents again knew what they were saying when they encouraged us to eat up our greens. Fresh vegetables provide us with so many essential vitamins and minerals that they must become a main part of our diet. Green vegetables also contain chemicals that allow our muscles and minds to relax. This reduces stress and refreshes our mind and body.

An area that we often overlook is the health of our blood. Most processed foods are highly acidic. So, by the way, is alcohol, smoking, sugar and pollution to name but a few. Research now suggests that our blood is healthiest when it is slightly alkaline. Eating your greens is a great way to alkalise your blood. Blood reaches literally every cell in our bodies and an acidic environment is a great place for diseases such as cancer to develop. Therefore, by eating alkalising foods, we are greatly increasing our chances of a disease free life. Here is a list of such foods –

Green cabbage	Lime
Spinach	Lemon
Leeks	Broccoli
Water cress	Tomato
Wheat grass	Carrot

Lettuce	Avocado
Parsnip	Turnip
Garlic	Celery

This is by no means an exhaustive list – all fruit and vegetables (especially raw) will have a positive effect here. In the list above is wheatgrass which is one of the most alkaline foods there are. If you go into a health food shop it is usually sold in bottles. It tastes like the bottom of a compost heap but I have found it sold with green tea which makes it more palatable. A good side effect is that it gives grey hairs back their colour. Worth a try then. A cheaper alternative is to squeeze half a lemon into some warm water and drink this. Although we think of lemon juice as acidic, it has an alkalising effect in our bodies. There are many good cook books with recipes that can make healthy food taste great. Another suggestion is to get a juicer and drink yourself healthy. Just to even things up here are highly acidic food and drink to avoid/ moderate –

Sugar	White bread
Canned foods	Beer
Red meat	Coffee
Processed foods	Black tea
Milk	Red wine
Butter	Fried foods
Cheese	Fats

Think for a moment of your body being like a battery. When a battery is working it is alkaline. As soon as the battery starts to breakdown it produces acid which sometimes oozes out of it. Our bodies are the same in that, as soon as we become acidic, we start to breakdown. The acid literally burns through our tissues causing damage. This makes us age, so if you eat your greens, you will look younger as well.

An excess of acid in the stomach can cause ulcers. Researchers now think that this acid also finds its way into the pancreas and damages the insulin producing cells. This can lead to Type 2 diabetes which shortens our life. No wonder this diabetes epidemic has coincided with an enormous increase of refined, sugar-filled food in our diets.

I have in my hand an article that leads with "Cancer is man-made say scientists." Scientists from Manchester University, England have made a study of hundreds of Egyptian mummies to test for signs of disease. As there were no surgical interventions available to remove tumours etc., they were surprised to find no evidence of any cancers in the remains. Furthermore Professor Rosalie David at the Faculty of Life Sciences has stated "There is nothing in the natural world that can cause cancer … so it has to be a man-made disease."

The Three White poisons

The advent of processed foods has coincided with the whole plethora of diseases and ailments that plague us today such as heart disease, high blood pressure, type 2 diabetes, obesity, cancer and arthritis.

We are the only species on the planet that messes with its own food and we are paying a heavy price – no pun intended there. The three foods to avoid here are white flour, sugar and salt. White flour is just wholemeal flour that has been bleached to make it look more attractive to eat. This bleaching process, however, kills all the nutrients originally in the grain. Furthermore, once digested, this "dead" food forms a gluttonous mass in our digestive system that is difficult to digest and usually finds itself adding to the fat around our midriffs. Refined sugar is responsible for the alarming rise in type 2 diabetes and obesity. When we ingest refined sugar our bodies over stimulates the pancreas to produce insulin in order to lower our blood sugar levels. This has the doubly tragic effect of overworking our pancreas until it eventually fails and also increases our blood pressure. Lastly, we do need salt in our diet and our blood is approximately 1% salt. The bad news, however, is that the average westerner gets up to 20 times the amount needed of this trace nutrient. Also table salt has anti-caking chemicals that are harmful. I take The Queen here as an example of someone who has no added salt in her food and seems to be doing OK.

Supplements

This is a contentious topic that divides opinion amongst the experts. In an ideal world we would eat the exact amount of nutritious food that our bodies need each day, but I fear few of us do. Furthermore modern farming methods have left the soil, in which our crops grow, in nutritional decline. For these reasons I take a good multi-vitamin and mineral supplement each day. This may be just psychosomatic and even if I don't need it the body will just get rid of any excess.

On a personal level I was diagnosed with asthma a few years ago and was given a steroid based inhaler to treat this condition. I researched for any natural remedies for this condition and discovered that this is another example of our bodies' immune system failing under the attack of modern pollution and household chemicals. An article I read recommended taking vitamin D3 and getting plenty of fresh air and doing these simple things has irradiated my symptoms. Do your research but I would encourage that you investigate and find natural cures to any conditions you have.

Sleep

It is no surprise that nowadays we get far less sleep (at least one hour) than people did fifty years ago. In an age of 24 hour information we push ourselves relentlessly and ignore our bodily signals with another cup of coffee.

Rest is essential if you are caring for someone so try to get 6 or 7 hours rest a night. It is thought that we were designed to sleep twice a day, the second sleep being more of a short snooze. If you can take a quick nap during the day it will do wonders for you.

Chronological age versus biological age

There is nothing we can do about our chronological age. This is due to how many days we have lived since we were born. We can, however, reverse our biological age by taking the necessary steps.

If we give ourselves rest, relaxation, healthy foods, exercise and plenty of water then the great gift of good health can be ours. The human body is remarkable in its ability to heal itself so we can undo a lot of damage by changing our health rituals.

Body Image

Going back to our main theme, there seems little doubt that the state of our body has a great effect on our image. We live in a body obsessed culture and we are constantly being bombarded with images of perfection through the media. We have to be aware of the effect on our self-esteem this has when we compare ourselves with often brush stroked images of "perfect people." We have to be comfortable with ourselves and set realistic targets on what we can achieve, given our age and busy lifestyles. Comparisons with people half our age are both unkind to ourselves and irrelevant. Eat well, exercise and enjoy life.

Here is a trick that I just picked up that helps you burn fat without dieting and exercise. It seems that there are two types of fat cells in our bodies. Just like there is good and bad cholesterol there are white fat cells and brown fat cells. Babies have a higher level of brown fat cells than adults. These cells contain a substance called mitochondria which generates body heat in young babies by burning white fat cells. In adults these brown fat cells appear to lie dormant but can be activated by hard physical activity.

These cells can also be activated to burn fat by cooling the body down. Have you ever noticed that if you get into cold water that after the initial shock it seems to warm up in a few moments. Obviously it is not the water that has warmed up, but your body has responded by burning fat to keep you warm. Rather than jumping into freezing water, the next time you take a shower gradually turn down the hot water until you allow 30 seconds of cold water to shower over you. Your brown fat cells are located in your chest, neck and upper back so this is all you need to cover. You will find this refreshing and it has other benefits such as detoxing your body, decreasing your blood pressure and strengthening your immunity. All at no cost in money and time!

I wish you the great gift of good health and now for the last part of integrity which is another massive and contentious subject …

SPIRIT

Albert Einstein referred to this as an "infinite intelligence." He realised that science could not explain many of the mysteries of life and the universe. Indeed the subjects of spirituality and religion have intrigued, obsessed and divided people for thousands of years. This is a controversial area but one that I think is vital for our integrity and our happiness.

Throughout history, people have drawn great strength through their beliefs and religious and spiritual organisations continue to do great work every day. I believe that everyone's beliefs should be respected and so I will now tell you what my thoughts are here. It does not mean I am right or wrong and it is not my intention or place to convert anyone to any particular philosophy. You can relax as you read this. That also applies to you atheists.

Firstly I see spirituality as a sense of connection to something greater than yourself. It is difficult to not stare at the night sky and not get a sense of awe and wonder, just as our ancient ancestors did. I always envy children in that they still see wonder and magic in all they do and it's time we reignited these wonderful feelings in ourselves. Whether you are an atheist, religious or spiritual let's all become child-like in our fascination with nature. We might just live longer, happier and more peacefully. Religion has the same sense of connection to this mysterious power and seeks to worship it. Often religion puts this power into a human form such as Jesus or God. The Dalai Lama explains God as being like a large mountain. He explains that the mountain (God) looks different depending from whichever direction you are looking. I think that is a great way of reconciling religious differences by realising we are looking at the same thing but from a different position. This great power you may wish to call God, God consciousness, Christ consciousness, Buddha, Allah or The Toa to name but a few. What matters is that your beliefs matter to you and benefits yourself and others.

I belief that we have all come from and are part of this great organising power. This power or energy is everywhere and nowhere. Confusing I know but think of gravity. It is an all powerful force in the universe that you cannot touch or see. It is nowhere but jump off a tall building and it suddenly appears. Scientists still have no explanation for gravity. We just need to know that this force exists even if we will never understand it.

I strongly believe there is a part of us which is spiritually perfect as we all come from perfection. Say out loud "I am spiritually perfect!" You can say that and feel good because it is true. At our core we are pure goodness and we are eternal. Whatever your beliefs are about the afterlife, we will all return back to our originating power. Whenever I think of my troubles, I try to remember that there is a spiritual part of me that is eternal, so how little they will matter in a million years.

OK, you are asking, then how do I explain all the stupid, thoughtless and often cruel things that people do? My favourite spiritual teacher is Dr Wayne Dyer who explains this brilliantly. He states that before we are born we trust totally in this power to provide everything we need to live. Then we are born and as we go from being a child to an adult we develop an ego which stands for Edging God Out. Instead of trusting in our maker we see ourselves as disconnected from everything and our focus turns on to ourselves. Our identity is therefore based on: 1. our possessions. We therefore define ourselves as how much we have. Our net worth becomes our self-worth. 2. Our body. This means that we only define ourselves as a living being and not a spiritual one. 3. Our accomplishments. We are only acceptable to ourselves and others if we have achieved x or done x.

This thinking defines our western society and leads, I believe, to most of the emotional and mental problems of our age. If we believe that we are defined purely by our possessions and we happen to lose everything, then we can see ourselves as being nothing. I think you will agree that this is not great for our happiness.

We are much more than our possessions, however nice they are. Also, if we only define ourselves as our body, then we are defining ourselves with something that declines over time. A much better idea is to recognise our human mortality, live healthily and appreciate that our eternal spirit will endure. I believe we are spiritual beings having a human experience.

The pressures we put on ourselves to achieve has given us our lifestyle, which is all well and good. We must also appreciate that we are spiritually whole and complete and we must appreciate the journey and not just focus on the destination. It is easy for our drive for success to become dissatisfied with our selves. If we allow our connection to God to strengthen us, then we approach our desires from a place of happiness and success becomes a pleasure. This increases our chances of success and raises our confidence.

Where do we find spirituality?

This is a great question. As humans we find we are naturally drawn to nature. We have forgotten that we are part of nature. For example, a spiritual person would never help destroy their environment, as to do so would be like drinking poison. We are connected and come from the same source as every living thing on the planet.

A walk in nature therefore, is a great way to reconnect with ourselves and our true essence. Most of us can watch water flow, or a fire burn, for hours. We also find trees and plants very soothing. This is because the shapes of nature are what is called fractal. This means that if you imagine a tree, it is both familiar in shape and simple. However, if you think of the leaves and bark, it also has infinitely complex patterns. This both soothes and fascinates the mind at the same time. No wonder people spend so much time in their gardens.

This feeling of connection will greatly affect how we view others. If we view everyone we meet as coming from the same source then we must all be one. Therefore everyone is our brother or sister. Imagine what that thought will do for our interactions with others and ultimately our feelings of connection.

Yes but who am I?

This is a question that scholars, philosophers and just about everyone else have puzzled upon for thousands of years. However, the majority of the human race seems no closer to answering this.

I believe that the answer is simply we are that which does not change. It is this eternal presence that we have talked about. It is the sacred place that is in us all.

From this idea we understand we are certainly not our life. Our lives are in a constant state of change. We are not our circumstances. We are not our thoughts either. Our thoughts never stop and constantly change as we gain knowledge, experiences and insights. We are not our emotions otherwise we would have to identify with the crazy rollercoaster we are all on.

Am I my body? Again you may have noticed that our bodies change somewhat as we age. I still regularly go to the gym looking for my twenty year old body. The trouble is I still come home with this old one.

This knowledge allows us to dissociate with all the above things. For example if my life is a "failure" then I am not. The "I" here being now who I really am. "I" can never be a failure as it is something eternal and perfect. It is separate from my life, body, possessions, finances, career, relationships, etc. All those things are temporary and only matter on the human level of consciousness. Who I truly am is what really matters.

In order to find out spiritual self, we need to take some of our attention out of our head and into our body. Just close your eyes and become aware of this inner space within you. I feel it in the solar plexus area. Often I ask myself: how do I know my spirit exists? This stills my mind and anchors me inside. It stops the mad chatter of my mind for a few moments.

This awareness brings you inner peace. It has been called many things. Jesus Christ called it the peace of God which transcends all understanding. Buddha referred to it as emptiness. Loa Tzu called it the Tao. It has been called the soul, inner peace, infinite intelligence, inner awareness and of course God. Karl Jung referred to it as the collective consciousness.

Think of your human existence as being on the horizontal plain. We are always grabbing at what we think will make us happy. We see happiness as being the next thing. The problem is the next thing will always only be just the next thing. (Think about that). We also always want to be in the next place, as that place always seems better than this place. This is one reason why the human race is always in a rush. The problem is that we miss out on the present moment, and the present moment is all we have.

Think of your spiritual existence as being on the vertical plain. If we give some attention to this inner place inside us, we stop our thoughts. If our thoughts are like clouds then we need to create a gap in them. When we become aware of this inner space we bring out the sun. This sun is our inner light which brings true happiness and peace. This is enlightenment, which is what Buddha described as the end of suffering.

I realise this subject is a bit heavy. If you want to go much, much deeper into this subject then I recommend reading "The Power of Now" by Eckhart Tolle. I found this book to be quite a challenge but it totally changed my whole outlook for the better. It was well worth the effort.

Meditation

How would you like to greatly improve your health by simply learning to relax? Humans have been meditating for thousands of years. All the research here seems to prove that regular meditation can improve your health, brain function, relieve stress and increase life expectancy. I had heard about this fact years before but I did not know where to start. Books I read on the subject made it sound so difficult and often linked the process to a certain religious belief. Finally I have come across an easy, effective way to meditate that is simple and fun.

It is known as "The release meditation." Firstly you will need some background music. I use a meditation track from YouTube. You can download a track from the internet or buy a CD. Next sit or lay down comfortably in a darkened room, not forgetting to minimise any distractions such as phone calls. Play the music softly and close your eyes. Then silently repeat the word release, release over and over. As you do this just focus your attention and energy in your inner body and breathing. As you do this you will be often interrupted by thoughts as we spend our entire lives inside our heads. No wonder we are all stressed. Just let your thoughts come and go as you focus inside and relax. This takes a little practice but soon you will love the experience. Twenty minutes is the optimum time that research has shown gives us the maximum results. Allow yourself the gift of deep relaxation for twenty minutes a day and you will be much more effective as a result.

Putting it all together

Here is a challenge for you. Why not commit to "The Hour of Power" every day for the next month? This involves 20 minutes of reading or studying, 20 minutes of exercise and 20 minutes of meditation. After 30 day you will feel great. Scientists have proved that after 30 days our brains create new neural pathways. This means that after 30 days any new actions form an almost unbreakable habit. It will be just like brushing your teeth and each day you will be strengthening your mind, body and spirit. You will take yourself to a new level.

OK this has been an important chapter and well worth a re-read. By strengthening our mind, body and spirit we are setting ourselves up for a long and happy life. What this book is about is change. This change has to start with ourselves. All compassion starts with self-compassion. You cannot like anyone more than you like yourself. Once we realise how incredible we are, we will see this in others and treat them accordingly. This information is to be absorbed slowly so that we can make the changes, we feel are needed, slowly over time. We must raise the consciousness of the world one mind at a time, starting with ourselves. How much better a place would the world be if there were no wars, no pollution, no crime and no poverty? That is a prize worth striving for.

Action Points

- List your top ten values – what do you stand for? Take the time to really define yourself and how you will live your life.
- From now on make all your decisions based on these values. This should lead to faster clearer

decisions which will make you more confident in yourself and in the eyes of others.

- Review your eating habits. Could you eat more alkalising foods? Could you replace white flour products with healthier wholegrain alternatives?
- Drink more water. Have a glass or bottle of water with you and continually take sips. You will feel increased energy and your skin will look younger.
- Get into exercise if you aren't already. Find something that is fun, gets you out of breath and does not hurt you. Join a club for extra motivation.
- Do the "cold shower" trick daily if you can. You will feel energised as you activate your body to burn fat.
- Practice your religion or spirituality. Feel your increased sense of wellbeing as you connect to a power that encompasses everything.
- Say to yourself "I am spiritually perfect" every day and you will know it is true.
- Do the release meditation once a day. Get back to knowing your happy, relaxed self.
- Commit to "The Hour of Power" for 30 days and be amazed at the results.

Now let's move on to the N in MINDSET. This makes life special and unique and stands for...

CHAPTER 3

NEW

"If you change the way you look at things, the things you look at change."- DR. Wayne Dyer

The speaker Bob Proctor often asks his audience the following question: When was the last time you did something for the first time? That question encapsulates the purpose of this chapter perfectly. Nothing will enhance our lives more quickly than trying something new. The problem is that we are very good at placing barriers up to stop us even trying. The good news is that the more we are willing to try something new the less we are worried about what others think. This gives our lives a sense of uncertainty. Again we all need a certain level of uncertainty to give life a different edge. Variety really is the spice of life. Trying new things also eliminates boredom from our lives.

Habits

Human beings are creatures of habit. Most of our day to day activities are automated to a great degree. This has the advantage of freeing up our minds to think through our daily challenges. The disadvantage is that it can take any variety, spice and fun out of our lives. Although we need a routine to be effective we need to bring in the power of NEW into our lives. This could mean –

NEW ideas.

NEW directions.

NEW thinking.

NEW relationships.

NEW attitudes.

NEW skills.

NEW career.

NEW challenges.

I once heard the writer Dennis Waitley say that habits are like submarines, in that they run silent and deep. This means it is easy to keep doing the same things which gives us the appearance of being stuck and we have all felt that particular frustration. In order to become unstuck we have to raise our sensitivity to see if any of our habits need improving or replacing entirely.

Turn Frustration In To Fascination

I was always one of those people who became quickly frustrated by technology, especially computers. I had convinced myself that I was a technophobe and pressing the 'on' button was as far as I could go to master my computer. I was actually indulging in two bad habits here. There first was getting frustrated in the first place. I think this stems in part with society expecting us to be instant experts at everything. The second bad habit was that by calling myself a technophobe to anyone who would listen I was labelling myself. All labels do is place self-limits on us.

What I try to do now is observe myself getting frustrated every time I have a technology meltdown. Instead of judging myself stupid in the moment, I just relax and watch myself getting hot under the collar. This has the effect of making myself laugh at my stupidity which lessens my stress and allows me to think through the problem. This has also enabled me to re-label myself as someone who is fascinated with technology and wants to constantly learn about it. I think this new habit of observing myself getting stressed and laughing about it has helped me make progress in many areas. We all need to stop taking ourselves too seriously as this can be counterproductive.

Time Management

This was another area I had challenges in so I decided to get fascinated with it. Most of us suffer from overwhelm and feel we do not have the time to do all that we have to in any 24 hour period. The Pareto principle states that 20% of our activities give us 80% of our results. I am sure you have heard of this but we often need reminding of the basics. In theory if we just concentrated on the vital 20%, we could work one day a week and be just as productive. The problem is that in a world full of distractions we often focus our energies on the trivial 80%. One way to get over this problem is to write out a MUST DO LIST and not a TO DO LIST. I have heard it said that we will always get our "musts" but we will rarely get our "shoulds." A good practice then, is to write out a must do list on a Sunday for the week ahead. Another good habit is to think on paper and not to start your week before it is finished on paper. This allows us to focus on what we need to accomplish and I find it satisfying to cross off tasks as they are completed. Also if you write down tasks in advance, it gives your subconscious mind time to consider the possibilities and come up with solutions. You can even label your tasks with an A, B or C. A being a "must do" task, B being a "should do" task and C being a "could do" task.

Eat that Frog

I have learnt a lot on this subject from Brian Tracy who is a master at productivity. Brian suggests that the first thing we should do every day is to "eat that frog." What he means by that is that if we have an unpleasant or difficult task to perform, we should tackle this first thing. This then frees you up to enjoy the rest of your day. We waste a lot of time worrying about things instead of just doing them. I have put a plastic frog on my desk at home to remind me of this.

The two main distractions in our days are emails and phone calls. An email is really just another person's agenda and may or may not be of any interest. I remember the days when you got a message that said: You've got email! Now, of course, it's more a case of please, please stop sending me all this junk. Most people are at the email overwhelm stage, so in order not to become its slave, I check my emails twice a day at set times. I use the scan and delete method whereby I instantly delete mail which is of no immediate interest, and scan read all the others. I then set aside a time where I respond to the remaining emails.

The trouble with phone calls is that they break your thought patterns and concentration. I am writing this book at home and when I write I have my mobile and landline on voicemail. I find if I can focus on one task at a time I am much more productive. Sorry ladies but research has shown that even you cannot multi-task effectively!

Money Management

This is a vital area that we all need to get a grip on. Physiologists state that we feel happy and effective in an area to the degree in which we feel we have control. This makes sense as a feeling of helplessness in any area hits our confidence and spills over to other areas of our lives. That said I want to give you a system of controlling your money which is simple and effective. You know by now that I like simple and this idea comes from Rohan Weerasinge.

First off you will need several accounts. The main idea of this system is that every penny you earn has a pre-defined purpose. All your monthly income is paid into your income account which will be your main checking bank account. Then you just set up a series of direct debits to your other accounts. These accounts will be called Living, Debt, Wealth, Fun, Education, Charity etc. This is where you need to sit down with your partner or spouse and agree what percentage of your income goes automatically into each account. This will of course depend on your goals and circumstances.

The purpose of the wealth account is to create long term prosperity. Even if you can only afford a small amount do not neglect to increase your wealth each month. This will give you a sense of power and confidence in your future. Most finance books recommend a minimum of 10% for investing but just start where you can. It is not the amount that is important but the habit of saving. We are building new habits here that empower us. The Fun account I view as a reward for the discipline of saving. A great way to reinforce this new habit is to take this money each month and indulge ourselves. You will not need my help thinking up ways to spoil yourself.

Many wealthy people emphasise the importance of charity or tithing as being fundamental to their wealth. The law of reciprocity states that what we give out comes back to us multiplied. The universe is an abundant place and you cannot out give it. When you give money away you are stating to the universe and to yourself that you have more than enough. This is abundant thinking and by thinking like this you will attract abundance into your life. It takes faith to give money away if you are struggling but generosity is a hallmark of a successful person. We must therefore be generous with our resources as this is true abundance. I am sure this resonates strongly within you.

Example Model

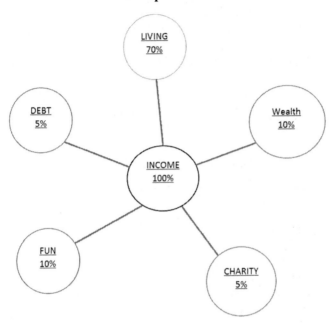

Certainty – Uncertainty

Tony Robbins states that there are six fundamental human needs. These are Significance, Connection/Love, Growth, Contribution, Certainty and Uncertainty. Whilst you will no doubt agree that the first four are fundamental to your life, the last two are a bit of a contradiction. Certainty is important to us as without it worry and anxiety creep in. It is good to feel certain that you will be paid at the end of the month, that your partner loves you and that we have a clean bill of health from the doctor. The problem comes when we have all our ducks lined up and we have total certainty in our lives. That problem is boredom. We have all heard reports of Hollywood stars who appear to have the complete package of looks, fame and fortune who are caught shoplifting or take an overdose. What they are seeking here is uncertainty. We all need variety, challenge and need for the unknown to stimulate us. This is where the need for something new in our lives is so important. This maintains our zest for life. Without uncertainty life becomes a monotonous cycle. This is why we like travelling to new places and countries.

I used to get frustrated when things did not work out as I wanted. Now I realise that how my life unfolds is meant to be a mystery. This is the real wisdom behind uncertainty. Enjoy the mystery.

Stress

There has been much written about the dreaded comfort zone. The problem is of course that we feel comfortable and safe in it which goes back to our need for certainty. We need to remind ourselves that every time we try something new we will feel uncomfortable. Instead of fighting this feeling, we just need to observe that it is there and appreciate it is a natural part of the change process. We all know that stress is a bad thing that can lead to illness if unchecked. Like cholesterol there is bad stress and good stress. This good form of stress is called eustress. "Eu" literally means healthy. Eustress is caused when we push beyond our limits and helps us to grow. Examples of eustress are the nerves you feel when you step up to deliver an important presentation or the feelings in your body if you push yourself in the gym. We need therefore to actively seek out eustress in our lives to build our confidence and self-esteem. Too much excitement can be a bad thing so just bring new things into your life at a pace you can handle. There is no rush if you know you are focused on the right path.

New Circumstances

So far we have been talking about new changes that we control. Unfortunately there are times when something new happens in our lives that is both unexpected and unwelcome. You may have heard the term "Black Swan Event" which refers to something happening that we just could not predict. These events are, in theory, highly unusual as the term suggests. This term was invented at a time that black swans were thought not to exist. The problem is that black swans have since been found in Australia and we all have experienced the unexpected. Every day people lose their jobs, get divorced and someone finds themselves looking after a sick relative. These occasions are the real test of our confidence. I believe that everything happens for a reason but it is difficult to know what it is when you are emotionally involved in the situation.

Often we cannot change what has happened but over time we can put a new meaning on it. I have heard it said that everything that gets in our way has been sent to help us.

Elizabeth Kubler-Ross wrote a famous book call "On Death and Dying" and in this book she wrote about the 5 stages we go through when we are facing death or any other major loss in our lives. This is often referred to as the DABDA model. The stages are –

1.   Denial
2.   Anger
3.   Bargaining
4.   Depression
5.   Acceptance

She states that we all must go through all or most of these stages before we can get to a state of acceptance of our loss. It is only through acceptance that we can find the strength to adapt to new circumstances. I suppose it's like the old saying goes: 'What doesn't kill you makes you stronger'. A lot of people have grown more in adversity than they ever would have if things had been easy. You can't make champions on a feather bed and often our problems are, in reality, opportunities in disguise. I suppose this uncertainty makes life so unique. We have all looked back at seemingly bad events and realised later that this was the best thing to happen to us. The quote at the start of this chapter tells us that once we alter our perceptions of our reality then our reality changes. Food for thought.

New Image

It is said that 90% of our opinion of someone is made in the first 7 seconds of meeting them. This should not be the case, but this is the reality. Appearances matter. Changing or improving our appearance then can have a dramatic effect on our influence on others and, in turn, our own confidence. The ladies reading this will agree that something magical happens when your hairdresser goes to work on you. You leave the salon walking a little taller, I am sure. We all feel more confident if we are dressed sharply. It is as if we subconsciously act according to our new look.

Corporations spend billions each year on brand image. Kentucky Fried Chicken changed to KFC, Federal Express to FEDEX and Nike is recognised worldwide by its swoosh logo. Pop stars and celebrities alike, spend fortunes on image consultants.

In the UK Tony Blair turned the old British Labour Party into New Labour and was duly elected into power. That subtle move changed the perception of an outdated party into one that was seen as modern and forward looking.

Affirmations

We must be willing to try anything that helps our progress. Affirmations are belief based statements that we say either out loud or to ourselves. They are most effective if you add a physical act to them. This drives the belief deeper into our subconscious mind. A positive emotion is also important here.

The next time you are walking down the street say to yourself repeatedly: "I feel confident." Smile as you do this and you will find your posture changes as you will walk taller. You can use this as you are about to give a presentation or in an important meeting.

Other affirmations I like are –

"I feel terrific"

"I like myself"

"I am unstoppable"

"I am healthy"

"I am wealthy"

"I am popular"

Liking yourself is vitally important because we cannot like anyone more than we like ourselves. Liking yourself makes you more loving, giving and likeable to others and strengthens our relationships. I practice these when I am working out or going for a walk. Positive self-talk is great as it shuts up that constant negative chatter that often goes on inside our head.

I must issue a note of caution here; affirmations without the appropriate action can mean we are deluding ourselves. This means if we affirm that we are healthy, we should at least put down the burger and fries and actually do something healthy.

The Habit of Gratitude

Expressing gratitude is also great for our self-image. Gratitude strengthens our appreciation of our lives and ultimately ourselves. When you wake up in the morning why not say to yourself "Thank you, thank you, thank you." We can only think one conscious thought at a time so the more positive thoughts we think, the less of the negative is going in.

Writing a gratitude list is powerful. Every day try to write one more thing you are grateful for. Remember to include all the great experiences, people and things from your past. It is also important to include all the great things that you will be, do and have in the future. This gives us a positive expectation of what is to come which heightens our optimism and excitement for the future.

We often criticise ourselves for not achieving all we intend to. We all have the habit of deleting our accomplishments from our minds and focusing on what we have not done. A useful thing to do, therefore, is to periodically write a victory list of everything that you have accomplished over a set period. This reviewing helps us appreciate just how far we have come. We should all take the time to smell the roses. This practice builds our sense of progress and renews our faith in ourselves. This leads us to be even more effective in the future.

You Lucky Thing

You have probably heard that luck is just an acronym for Labouring Under Correct Knowledge. The truth is that luck is not something that just happens to us, but is something we can influence through our actions. The more new disciplines, subjects and approaches we get involved in, the luckier we will be. People around you will be surprised at your change in fortune when in fact life is often just a numbers game. The more things we try the more likely we will discover new talents and abilities that we did not know we possessed.

Professor Richard Wiseman wrote a book called "The Luck Factor" which was the result of interviewing over 1,000 people to find out why some people appear luckier than others. He came up with 4 luck principles which I list below:

Principle 1 – Lucky people create, notice and act upon the chance opportunities in their lives.

N.B. It appears these people build a strong "network of luck" by networking with as many new people as possible. They have a relaxed attitude about life and are always open to new experiences.

Principle 2 – Lucky people make successful decisions by using their intuition and gut feelings.

N.B. Not only do lucky people listen to their intuition but they take steps to boost it. This is done by listening to what our feelings are telling us.

Principle 3 – Lucky people's expectations about the future help them fulfil their dreams and ambitions.

N.B. Lucky people see their good luck as natural and expect it to continue in the future. They persevere to achieve their goals in the face of great difficulties and failures. They expect their interactions with others to be lucky and successful.

Principle 4 – Lucky people are able to transform their bad luck into good fortune.

N.B. lucky people always see a positive side to their bad luck. They are convinced that any ill fortune will always work out for the best. Lucky people do not dwell on their bad fortune. They know that the darkest hour is always before the dawn.

My thanks to Professor Wiseman for giving us such a great insight into the much misunderstood concept of luck. We now have 4 great ideas for increasing our luck in the future. This leads to a new sense of optimism, happiness and confidence in ourselves and our lives.

Luck is really just another word for chance so we should be looking at luck as a scientific principle. Just like a professional gambler has a system in place that ensures he or she is always lucky, we can ensure our own luck by incorporating these 4 principles into our lives. Wiseman has a series of tests in his book, one being your "Luck Profile" which I have included for you to score yourself with.

Your Luck Profile

Score each of the following statements as follows:-

1.   Strongly disagree
2.   Disagree
3.   Uncertain
4.   Agree
5.   Strongly agree

Just write down your first answer you think of to the following questions –

1.   I sometimes chat to strangers when queuing at a supermarket or bank.
2.   I do not have a tendency to worry and feel anxious about life.
3.   I am open to new experiences such as trying new types of food and drink.
4.   I often listen to my gut feelings and hunches.
5.   I have tried some techniques to boost my intuition such as meditation or just going to a quiet place.
6.   I nearly always expect good things to happen to me in the future.
7.   I tend to try and get what I want from life even if the chances seem slim.
8.   I expect most of the people I meet to be pleasant, friendly and helpful.
9.   I tend to look on the bright side of whatever happens to me.
10.   I believe that even negative events will work out well in the long run.
11.   I don't tend to dwell on things that haven't worked out well for me in the past.
12.   I try to learn from the mistakes that I have made in the past.

Don't worry if your score is low as it just means you have plenty of room for improvement. Just keep the luck principles in mind and try to live them for a month and watch your score rise. These are new concepts but just a little progress will do wonders. Any score over 40 out of a total of 60 is pretty good.

Action Points

•   Is there a new skill or hobby that you would like to try?

•   Realise that every time you feel uncomfortable doing something new that this is good. You are pushing out of your comfort zone and experiencing 'eustress' (good stress).

•   Write out a list of affirmations and link an appropriate action to each one as you repeat them.

•   Write out a list of everything you are grateful for. Add to it over time and feel good when you refer to it.

•   Do you need to accept a loss in your life? Acceptance will help you to lessen the pain and move on.

•   Write out a list of everything you have accomplished over the last month. Celebrate your victories however small. Treat yourself to something nice.

•   Apply the 80/20 principle and see how it makes you more effective in managing your daily tasks.

•   Work out your luck factor. Realise that as you practice the 4 luck principles your luck must improve. The professor says so.

I trust you realise by now the importance of the word new. There is great wisdom in uncertainty as it gives us growth, excitement, variety and freedom from boredom. We have covered a lot here so, as always, just let the changes come into your life slowly.

In the next chapter we discuss something that is vital to do in order to get the most out of life. We must remember, therefore, to always ...

CHAPTER 4

DREAM

"Whatever the mind can conceive and believe, it can achieve" – Napoleon Hill

I firmly believe that happiness equals progress. With this in mind then we need to constantly find new ways to enhance our progress and our lives. I am talking about the subject of goal setting. If you have never set goals before, then I think you will find this chapter a real eye opener. All successful people have clear goals which stretch them to reach new heights. If you are new to this then don't worry as, with everything else in this book, just start slowly and simply enjoy the benefits.

Brian Tracy is famous for saying that goals are everything and everything else is just commentary. As this is such an important subject, let's explore this subject in depth.

Goals are stated intentions about what we intend to be, do or have. They are best written down as a constant reminder as to where our focus should be.

Why Set Goals?

If you have a set of goals written down then congratulations. Only 3% of people do, which again leaves 97% pretty much trusting to luck. If you have goals, I would suggest that you get them out and relook at them, as this subject has developed over the last few years.

In our modern world most people are dabblers. With a million and one distractions to eat up our time it is very difficult to focus. As we discussed earlier, clear goals allow us to focus on the critical few and to ignore the trivial many. It is easy to major in minor things and goals allow us to focus our time and energy.

There is a part of the brain called the Reticular Activating System or RAS. The RAS tells our conscious brain what to notice as we would be overwhelmed otherwise. Setting clear goals allow us to train this part of the brain to notice anything that relates to our goal. For example, if you want to go on holiday then your brain tends to notice all the information around you that relates to this. The problem is that we use this skill on a random basis to get our desires met. Written goals are like a contract with our brains to notice only the things that matter. Albert Einstein was once asked for his phone number by a reporter who wanted to interview the scientist. Einstein replied that he did not know it as he did not need to, but knew where it was written down. Einstein was so focused on discovering the laws of the universe that he let nothing else in to his mind. Talk about focus!

Why Don't People Set Goals?

I think there are many reasons for this and just a few are:-

- Goal setting is not taught in our school system.
- People therefore do not know how to set goals.
- It is not considered socially acceptable or "normal"
- People are afraid they will fail to reach their goals.
- People are afraid they will be laughed at.
- People think that it is hard work and painful.
- People think they lack the discipline to persevere with them.

This is quite a list and is certainly not exhaustive. There are many other reasons but it only takes one. Ignorance is a problem but that can easily be overcome by reading this chapter. If you are focused and goal driven then you may get laughed at for not being normal. By definition the 3% who have goals will be considered weird. That is a small price you may have to pay. Just remember, what other people think is their business. We are talking here about your happiness which is far more important. You may just want to keep your goals private rather than be burdened with someone else's negativity.

The reason people link pain to goals is that we often just set New Year resolutions. Often we focus on what we don't want. For example, I must get out of debt or I must lose this weight. They are about disciplining ourselves and so we don't get too excited about them. This lack of energy is the main reason most people have given up within 9 days. The solution is to therefore focus on what we want and let our goals inspire us. Let's face it – none of us need motivation to eat our favourite dessert. Goals have to be attractive or else they will not attract us.

A great goal and a great life

Andrew Carnegie arrived in America in 1848 as a penniless migrant from Scotland. He became the first great industrialist the country produced and also the world's richest man. It is said that when he died, his assistant was clearing out his desk when they found an old, yellowed piece of paper. On this paper was written "I will spend the first half of my life making money and the second half giving it all away." This was written when Carnegie was a teenager. Today his Carnegie Institute gives away millions of dollars every year to worthy causes. What a great example of a goal that has lived on after his death. This is the power of goals.

Tony Robbins says that we need to create a compelling future. People give up and sink into depression if they lose hope. We need goals and a vision that pulls us effortlessly towards our future, because it is so compelling. OK, that said, let us move on to the mechanics...

How to Set Goals

There are dozens of books on this subject which can contradict each other. The most commonly used goal setting technique is the SMART model. The acronym stands for –

Specific

Measurable

Achievable

Realistic

Timed

Examples of SMART goals would be –

"By 1st January 2015 I will own a black BMW 318i series with black leather seats."

"On my 50th birthday I will have a net worth of one million US Dollars."

The above goals fit the formula. Being specific about what you want certainly helps and the act of writing them down is like a formal contract with yourself. This greatly increases your chances of success.

The latest research, however, points out a few problems with this model. This technique was developed in the 1970s and science has advanced somewhat since. You probably know that the mind is divided into the conscious and the subconscious mind. This is also referred to as the unconscious mind. The conscious mind is the (mostly) rational and logical thinking part of the brain. This conscious part is used to set our goals. The conscious mind responds to logic and adheres to Newtonian physics. In other words it understands the world we live in and concepts such as time, distance, etc.

One example of conscious thinking would be: "I need to travel from London to Edinburgh by car. The distance is 500 miles so at an average speed of 50 MPH it will take me 10 hours. This is how we plan out the multitude of tasks we do each day.

The subconscious mind is much more powerful than the conscious and has until now, been shrouded in mystery. The subconscious does not respond to logic but purely responds to emotion. It cannot discern what is real from what is not. It can only accept information fed to it by the conscious mind. It cannot reject information like our conscious mind can. It also adheres to quantum physics. This means that it does not understand the concept of time or indeed distance. In quantum physics particles can disappear and reappear somewhere else in <u>no time!</u>

Before we get too heavy I must confess that I don't really understand much of this. What is important here is that we know that these things work and leave how they work to the experts. It is not necessary to understand how your computer works, but only that it does. That is unless you are one of those people who has to know how everything works. I am certainly not one of those people, but without you guys, I suppose science would not advance.

We also now know that the subconscious only responds to the first person and does not understand negative commands. Therefore we need to change "On the 1st January 2015 I will never smoke again" to "I am a non-smoker." The second goal is written in the first person, the present tense (I am) and states that I am something (a non-smoker in this example.)

If we revisit our previous SMART goals they now read –

"I own a black BMW 318i series with black leather seats."

"I have a net worth of one million US dollars."

We use the conscious mind to set our goals. Where the subconscious is vital is in the attainment of our goals. The trick here is to become effective at communicating with the subconscious mind to achieve our goals. This is done through emotion and positive visualisation. With the first goal then we need to visualise with feeling the black BMW. We need to feel the leather seats, the pride and excitement of driving the car, the salesman handing the keys over to us etc. etc. The more emotion you put into this the better. Also imagine using all your senses to experience the sound of the engine, the sights involved, the feel and smell of the seats and you can even taste the success!

Goal setting should be fun so we need to become childlike and really fire our imagination. Albert Einstein once said that imagination is more powerful than knowledge. It is time to re-connect with this power.

After we have visualised our goals as already having happened, we should be grateful. Gratitude is a purely positive emotion and in this state we are telling our subconscious that it is already creating our desired outcome.

Scientists have talked a lot about the fact that we live in an uncertain universe. With this in mind we need to detach ourselves with how we achieve the goal and just allow the subconscious to work its magic. All we need to do is just keep a clear vision in our minds of what we want and keep feeding our subconscious with this vision.

We also need to detach ourselves from the desired outcome. We need to stay relaxed, focused and be open to an even better outcome. In the BMW example if you were offered a better model for the same price you would not worry that you had "failed" in your goal. A smaller goal can lead to something bigger and we want to be open to receiving more than we asked for.

Lastly we need to take massive action. Just do everything you can to bring this goal into reality. Go to the car dealership and ask for a test drive, look at the colour brochures, negotiate a great deal and earn the extra money needed. Do whatever it takes and if it does not work then just change your strategy. We need to be flexible in how this goal will materialise.

To recap goal setting –

1.   Decide on your why. What are the benefits of achieving this goal? Create a burning desire that will attract the necessary resources, people and circumstances that will bring your goal into reality.

2.   Use your conscious mind to set and write your goals in the present tense, first person and be as specific as you can.

3.   Use your subconscious mind by visualising, with emotion the desired outcome. Do this as often as possible.

4.   Be grateful for your goal as this greatly increases your chances of success. It is already happening.

5.   Detach yourself from how this goal will happen. Trust in your subconscious to provide exactly what you want.

6.   Detach yourself from the precise outcome. Something better might show up!

7.   Take massive action and be infinitely flexible in your approach.

Let your heart rule your head

You probably think that I got the above title back to front. We have been trained to only trust our rational minds and not our gut feelings. You only have to look at the state of the world to realise where this has got us. Seriously though, we need to really listen to those moments of intuition and not suppress them. This is the subconscious talking to us and we need to take notice.

This intuition is usually a feeling of certainty or of being compelled to act. We have activated our subconscious through visualisation and now we must trust it to guide us to our desired outcomes. Just go with the flow and allow the wisdom of uncertainty into your life.

Women are more attuned to this than men. It is the feeling that something just does or does not feel right. Whether this is because women are more in touch with their feelings I am not sure. We men need to cultivate this more and appreciate that our feelings are compelling us to act. The word emotion originates from the verb to move. There is motion in emotion so let's be "moved to act." As often is the case, our lifetime of conditioning around this subject is just plain wrong.

Another time we can use the subconscious to problem solve is just before you go to sleep. Just think of a problem you have and ask for the solution. Say to yourself "I wonder what I should do about ......" Then in the morning as you wake up you may get an insight into your problem. This is your subconscious giving you a solution. This takes a little practice but why not allow this power to work for you whilst you sleep? This is why I said in the last chapter, a good idea to write out your must do list on a Sunday. This allows your subconscious to get to work on solutions in time for Monday morning.

You can get these intuitive flashes at any time. Newton was under an apple tree when the idea of gravity came to him. Einstein was sick in bed when the theory of relativity first entered his mind. The theory of displacement came to Aristotle when he was in the bath. We have all had good ideas when going for a walk or taking a shower. It is time we acted on them.

What Goals Should I set?

The answer to this question is quite simple. We should set goals in all the areas that are important to us. I set goals in eight key areas which are –

HEALTH

How can we do well if we don't feel well? We need a level of energy and a feeling of vitality to enjoy life. Some goals can be measured, such as an income goal, whilst other goals are life goals that need daily attention.

Our health needs daily maintenance as we never want to stop feeling healthy. As we have discussed, just set out a health plan and make steady progress. Remember that happiness equals progress.

My health goal is "I AM HEALTHY." I then have written down a plan to maintain this which changes with time and as I learn more in this area.

RELATIONSHIPS

Psychologists estimate that 80% of our happiness comes from our relationships with others. Conversely 80% of our unhappiness also comes from our interactions with others. We have all felt the stress of a bad relationship and there is nothing more painful. We are social animals and in prison the most feared punishment is solitary confinement. Remember that we cannot like anyone more than we like ourselves, so our relationship with our self needs exploring too. The affirmation "I like myself" is vital here as this raises our self-esteem which, in turn, improves our interactions with those around us.

One of my goals is "I ENJOY GREAT RELATIONSHIPS." You can set family goals here and also goals for your intimate relationship. It is said that you cannot spend "quality time" with someone but only time. Cultivate this area and feel the benefits in terms of your happiness and of those that are closest to you.

WEALTH

If the word wealth bothers you then you can change it to abundance. We live in an abundant universe. Everything is just energy and that goes for money. If we use money wisely then it is a force for good. Indeed it is said that 90% of relationship break ups are, in part at least, caused by money issues. This reason alone is enough to convince us that we need to take action and set goals in this area. True wealth is being happy with what you have got.

My goal here is simply "I AM WEALTHY." Money is just a side effect of what we do. The late Jim Rohn once gave this piece of advice: "Be happy with what you have got whilst you pursue all you want". I think this is a great insight into living a contented life.

CONTRIBUTION

Brendon Burchard, in his book *The Charge*, says that we will ask ourselves three questions at the end of our lives –

1.   Did I live?
2.   Did I love?
3.   Did I matter?

It is the third question that contribution addresses. Caring for others is one of our greatest drives and gives our lives true meaning. No one will remember us for what material possessions we had. All that they will remember is what we did for others. The real heroes of our society are the people who care for and contribute to others. Often this is done with little or no recognition. Remember it is how we feel about ourselves that matters and not what others think. We can contribute our time, our work and our money. Most of us can get a sense of contribution through our work. Often we think of work as something we just have to do to pay the bills. Doing a great job makes us feel good about ourselves and contributes to both our company and our family through job security.

One of my goals here is: "I CONTRIBUTE TO OTHERS."

PURPOSE

This is the most exciting area to set goals in but it can take a bit of thought. Napoleon Hill stated that we all need a major definite purpose in life. This will usually be your life's passion and may not be accomplished in your lifetime. It could be a legacy you want to leave behind such as a foundation. It does not matter what it is.

To truly discover what your passion is, ask yourself this question: What would I do if money was not an issue to me? You may be in the fortunate position where your work is your passion because you would continue to do it for free. This is great as this can also be how you contribute as well. If you are a priest, teacher or a doctor then you probably have your life's purpose.

This chapter is about dreaming so what would you do, be or have? Would you travel the world, work for your favourite charity or play the guitar all day? Life, as they say, is not a dress rehearsal so we all need a purpose that inspires us.

My goal here: Well I am not telling you all my secrets.

LIFESTYLE

This area is all about how we live our lives. Regardless of our circumstances we can make small changes here that can create a big difference. This is about focusing on the quality of our life and not just on our standard of living. This can include our living environment. We can often brighten our mood just by cleaning, tidying up a mess or redecorating a room. We don't need to spend a fortune, as just a bunch of flowers in a vase can transform a room and our sense of well-being.

We covered a lot of this ground in the last chapter, when we discussed bringing in new habits and experiences into our lives where possible. This acts as a pattern interrupt in our thinking which can give us a mental lift.

My goal here: "I CREATE MY IDEAL LIFESTYLE."

PERSONAL GROWTH

This is where we reconnect with the fun of learning. Children love to learn and have a natural curiosity. It is frightening how quickly they learn to walk, talk and develop. They are learning machines. Nothing will stop them from mastering a skill. They will try over and over again until they succeed. They seem to have no fear of failure. I have heard it said that if humans did not learn to walk until they were thirty, most of us would still be crawling on our backsides! Most of us would give up as soon as we fell over a couple of times and bumped our knees. As soon as our friends laughed at us we would want to give up. A child will attempt to walk until he or she succeeds. They are totally focused on their goal and could not care less what others think. We can learn a lot from kids.

Nothing stands still in the universe. If we are not growing and moving forward then we are going backwards.

My goal here: "I constantly grow."

MINDSET

To maintain a happy, positive, goal-directed attitude we must think happy, positive goal directed thoughts. The goal behind all goals is happiness. This is truly the goal of goals. In view of this happiness is our number one priority and what this whole book is about.

If my goal is to get that black BMW, what I really want is the feeling when I get the car. What is that feeling? A sense of pride, a feeling of accomplishment, a feeling of being a winner. This of course contributes to my ...HAPPINESS.

Just bear this in mind when you set your goals. All human action is driven by our need to go from pain to pleasure. Our ultimate goal is the happiness of ourselves and those closest to us. The problem is that our consumer driven culture has lied to us about what makes us truly happy. Happiness lies within us. Nothing outside of ourselves will ever make us happy. Just imagine that I had my BMW. After my initial euphoria and pride I would return to my previous level of happiness. After all it is just a car. I will then need another object to make me happy. This is why "shopaholics" are never satisfied. Can you see how this lie works? Finding out what does not give us long term happiness is just as valuable as what does. There will be a lot more on this subject to come.

My goal here: "I have peace of mind."

A Major definite Purpose

It does not matter how many goals you have. Often it is best to start with a small goal such as "I will go to the cinema next Tuesday." Start where you can and gradually develop this skill. If you go through the process and complete a small goal it will give you the trust and confidence in the system. This is not a race or competition so go at a pace that suits you.

As stated earlier, when you have your list of goals you need to pick one that is your major definite purpose. This goal could well be your main purpose in life. This is the one goal that you must be, do or have. It is your number one focus and priority. This one goal gives your life direction and meaning. This goal can, of course change with time. It is your number one goal.

But I need a deadline!

My system goes against conventional goal setting wisdom in that I do not give myself deadlines. My thinking here is that if I want something so much then why do I need a deadline? You can have deadlines in your planning to achieve your goals. For instance your goal might read "I am my ideal weight." You can then have a plan to: 1. Find out what your ideal weight is, by say consulting with your doctor. 2. Work out how much weight you need to lose – say 28 pounds. 3. Set a realistic deadline to lose the weight. Let's see – that's 392 ounces so that would be 4.35 ounces a day for 90 days. 4. Take action to bring this goal into reality.

This goal suggests to me that after you have hit your ideal weight you will <u>maintain</u> it. We don't want to hit our target and then start bingeing. What we are after is slow but permanent change. We don't want some crazy yo-yo diet. Just as an aside, we don't want to lose weight – we want to release it. What we lose we subconsciously try to find or replace. If I say that I have lost my pen then I either want to find it or get another one. We don't want the excess weight coming back, so we just intend to release it.

Be careful what you wish for

I once heard a story of a woman who attended a goal setting workshop. She decided to write a goal to attract her ideal man. She made a complete description of this man and stated that he was between five feet, ten inches and six feet in height. One year later she met the trainer of the workshop with her new husband. The trainer congratulated her on her success and then noticed that the husband had a built up shoe on his left leg. It turns out that he is 6 feet tall if he stands on his right leg and 5 feet 10 if he stands on his left. This supposedly true story indicates that we get exactly what we wish for. The moral here is to word our goals carefully!

Who should I tell about my goals?

I have shared some of my goals with you to show you how to word them. As you are reading this book we are like- minded in that we both want progress in our lives. It is up to you who you share your goals with. I tend to keep my goals private as I don't need the negativity of other people. Change frightens other people around you as it can be unnerving to them. The people around you have their own concept of you and you are ruining this by changing yourself. I only share my goal with someone I feel is genuinely interested in helping me attain it. We are not trying to change the world, just ourselves. If your nearest and dearest family see changes, and comment on this, then you can educate them if they are open to this. People only change if they want to, so don't force this.

Often we do need the support of family and friends to attempt a goal. One powerful reason to set goals is other people. If we can show others how our goals benefit them, they will be more inclined to help.

Think small

My advice, as always, is to gain momentum by starting with small goals and build up slowly. Some goals are easily measured, i.e. weight loss. Others, such as happiness, are subjective as how happy can we be? We can have a mixture of measurable or objective goals along with subjective goals.

We can then build up to larger goals. These are the goals that are compelling and excite us with hope and expectation of what is to come. Andy Harrington says to make our goals so big that our problems seem insignificant. This is great advice, as goals keep our minds on what we want.

Do you think goals affect our attitude? Of course. Someone who has clear goals has a sense of urgency and purpose. It shows in how they walk, how they talk and in their handshake. Attitude is everything. Our attitudes are contagious in that they affect everyone we come into contact with. We need to have an attitude that is worth catching. Goals give us a sense of being a winner and we all want to win. We just need to decide and define what winning means to us. There is no stereotype for success. Success is not a black BMW!

DO I need a daily ritual?

A lot of the books I have read advise reading your goals out loud every morning and evening, along with visualising them. This is good advice if you can do it. I tend to have my goals with me and look at them when I can. The problem I find with strict rituals is that it feels like hard work. I want my goals to be fun and to inspire me to take action. You may want to start reading your goals out loud once or twice a day to start with to "cement" them into your mind.

Another idea to really focus your mind, is to write your goals out each day. If you write them out in block capitals this requires greater concentration than your normal writing. This has the effect of burning your goals deeper into your subconscious.

Another idea I picked up somewhere is to write your goals on cards. Cut the cards into credit card sizes and put them into a credit card wallet. This is a good idea because it keeps your goals private but enables you to take them out of your handbag or pocket and refer to them often. You can read them at lunchtime, or any spare moment, and quietly visualise them. People will just think you are having a nap.

Some people have their goals on their screen saver at home. Some people put their goals on a wall or on their bedside table. Another idea is to create a dream board. This is where you download or cut out pictures and place images of what you want to achieve onto a wall board or an online document. This is good as it gives you a clear mental target to aim for.

Just have fun playing and experimenting and you will soon find what works for you.

ACTION POINTS

- Decide the areas of your life that you want to set goals in. If you are not sure then take a look at your values, as they are your best guide as to what you want.

- Don't worry if you can only think of one or two. The fact that you realise you don't know what you want is a big breakthrough. Most people don't even know that they don't know want they want in life.

- Start with a small goal(s) to test your new skills.

- Ask yourself why you want to be, do or have this goal? Is it just a wish or preference? All goals have a cost in terms of effort, time or money. Are you willing to pay the price?

- Set your goal in writing using the first person, first tense. For example, "I have... I own... I am... "

- Run each goal through the 7 step process.

- Take immediate action of your goal, however small.

- Make plans to achieve your goals, but allow your subconscious mind to provide as many options as possible.

- Above all have fun. This is your chance to be a child. This is like your present list to Santa Claus so treat yourself.

This chapter was about giving ourselves clear objectives and direction in our lives. Your goal can be to improve an existing area of your life. Some people score each area of their life from 1 to 10 and set goals where they have the lowest score. Just do what feels right and experiment a little. Bear in mind that the longer the period between setting a goal and taking action, the less likely we are to achieve our goals or even start them. Procrastination really is the thief of time.

In the next chapter we will explore another area that is vital to ensure our long term happiness. In order to achieve this we must control our...

CHAPTER 5

STATE

"Your success and happiness lies in you. Resolve to keep happy, and your joy and you shall form an invincible host against difficulties." – Helen Keller

Have you ever done something where you surprised yourself? Either good or bad? It was all to do with the state you were in at that moment. If we are in a highly resourceful state then we can call upon our resources to handle any situation. Conversely, if we are in a fearful, stressed or depressed state then often our results are disappointing.

The purpose of this chapter is to realise that, regardless of what is happening around us, we have the ability and power to manage our states. Our states are caused by our emotions as a result of our thoughts and actions, often being triggered by events. Another word for describing our state is simply our mood. These events or stimuli are created internally or are the result of external events.

Any one of a multitude of things can change our state or mood in a heartbeat. We have all felt great one moment and then lousy the next. We are often to be found on an emotional rollercoaster which leaves us exhausted at the end of the day.

I would like to show you the following diagram which is a model from the science of NLP. Our brains are, of course, staggeringly complicated and this model simplifies and helps us understand what causes our states.

The NLP Communication Model

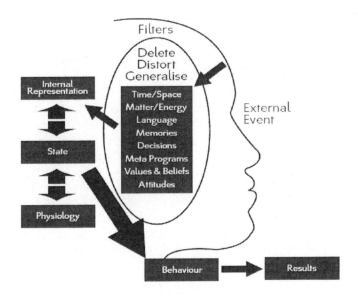

It is estimated that our nervous systems are bombarded with up to 10 million pieces of information per second! If we noticed everything then our brains would go into total overload and meltdown in a couple of seconds. Because of this our subconscious mind filters all this information. It does this as in the above model, by filtering, distorting and deleting information that it thinks the conscious mind does not need.

Our conscious minds can only handle between 5 and 9 pieces of information at a time. This information is coming to us through what we see, hear, touch, smell and taste.

Most of this information is <u>deleted</u> as irrelevant. There are millions of nerve receptors in our bodies constantly firing signals to our brains. We do not need to know what each one is feeling and doing, so they get deleted.

<u>Generalising</u> information is useful as this simplifies our lives. For instance we generalise how doors, cars and most everyday objects work so that we do not have to learn these skills every day. This has obvious benefits. The problem is that our generalisations can be inaccurate or inappropriate. For instance a generalisation about a particular race or age group can cloud our judgements.

Have you ever said anything to someone that they took offence to? It left you confused as that was not your intention at all. This was because they <u>distorted</u> your words due to their particular filters. This gave your words a completely different meaning.

We create our own reality

Everyone is applying these three filters all the time. Because we are all different, our brains are deleting, distorting and generalising differently. This is due to many factors, such as –

Age
Experiences
Attitude
Politics
Religious beliefs
Values
Memories
Internal language

This means that all of us are experiencing our own version of reality. We create an internal representation or perception of reality. In other words we give every experience a meaning. This means that if you gave a talk to one hundred people you would, in reality, deliver one hundred different talks! No wonder the human race is so screwed up.

We literally create our own universe through our thoughts. Now you know why it often feels as if nobody understands you, and vice versa! The psychologist Karl Jung said that perception is projection. What this means is that we project our perception of reality, both to ourselves and also to the outside world, through our reactions or behaviours.

This perception or internal representation results in our state. Our perception causes us to give this event a meaning. If we think that this situation is bad then we get angry or stressed. If we perceive the same situation as good then we get excited or happy. Can you see now why two people can react very differently to the same situation? That was a little heavy but this all leads to the following important conclusions –

- No one experiences reality.
- We only experience our perception of reality.
- We create our own reality.
- We all live in our separate realities.
- Every event that made us unhappy is an illusion!

This is quite a revelation to you, I am sure. The state we are in then dictates our behaviour, which leads to our results. If a situation makes us angry then we act appropriately (or inappropriately). If the same situation makes us laugh then we will probably act in a totally opposite way.

Can you see how this information can help us in our lives to manage our states to produce better results? OK, so now you know what causes our states then we need to know how to better manage them. This is best achieved through our physiology.

Physiology is the key

Imagine if you were walking down the high street and someone went skipping past you with a great big silly grin on their face. Would you think "There goes another depressed person in the world" or rather "I want whatever they are on!"

I am guessing it might be the latter and this gives us a great clue to managing our states.

As the diagram suggests there is a big link to how we use our body and our emotional state. For instance, how would you expect a depressed person to stand? Slumped or upright? How would they breathe? Shallow and fast or slow and deep? Where would they look? Down or up? Would their movements be fast or slow?

A depressed person does not consciously adopt a depressed position so that we can all see that they are depressed. It is not a legal requirement for them to act that way.

What happens is that their perception of the world is that there is no hope so they behave in a depressed manner (expressed through their physiology) which gives them the result of being depressed.

The takeaway here is that we do our emotions through our physiology.

Let's manage our state

I apologise if that section was a little complex. I think though, that time spent learning how we think is time well spent. The purpose of this book is to give us the tools to increase our sense of wellbeing. It is not meant as a judgement on others. People with clinical depression still need professional help and advice. This book is not some miracle cure but just a practical guide to assist where it can. As I have stated several times, change takes time so this is about increasing our awareness. Little changes over time equal big results.

Breathing

We all have coping strategies for dealing with our day to day stresses. Some of our strategies are good and others not. To repeat a previous example, you probably see people outside buildings smoking a cigarette. The smoker believes that the act of smoking is calming them down. The real reason they are now feeling calmer is that they are taking in the deep breaths that their body craves.

The smoker, however, has made an association in his own mind that it is the cigarette that calms him or her down. This shows how powerful our minds are in playing tricks on us. Nicotine is a powerful stimulant that can easily double our heart rate. This is the opposite of calm.

If you are stressed or anxious then you can bet that your breathing is shallow and high in your chest. You can slowly do ten in breaths to the count of ten followed by ten out breaths to the same count. This way you are breathing deeply and from the stomach. This gives your body what it needs: oxygen. Alternatively go for a walk. This is why exercise relaxes us. It clears our mind and allows us to think more clearly. This won't solve the problem but it will put us in a more resourceful state to deal with it.

All these strategies are designed to help us cope a little better with our day.

Vision

I was amazed to learn that we can change our state with our eyes alone. There are two types of vision: foveal and peripheral.

Foveal vision is where we focus on a single point that is often close to us. When you are threading a needle you are in foveal. Staring at a computer screen also causes us to be in foveal vision. The problem with this is that it is stressful and tiring. This is why we need to take regular breaks if we use a computer often. The next time you are feeling worried or depressed you can bet that you are in foveal vision. You will be looking down and focused on a particular point.

For example, the other day I was filling up my car with petrol (gas if you are American). For some reason I tend to focus on the top of the pump as I fill up.

This has put me into foveal vision. Suddenly I start to moan to myself about the cost of the petrol and then the cost of everything and then that I have not had a pay rise …etc. etc. After a minute of moaning and getting myself into a bad mood, I broke this thought pattern by just looking up and relaxing my eyes.

Try this the next time you start to feel bad.

Peripheral Vision

Whenever you look up, or straight ahead and relax, you are in peripheral vision.

A good example of this is again driving. When you first learn to drive you are often nervous. Because of this the driver will often focus on the front of the car and therefore be in foveal vision. No wonder our driving lessons were so tiring.

As we become more confident drivers, we start to relax and we go into peripheral. This means that we notice the cars in the opposite lanes without having to move our head. We have a wide field of vision in this state.

Have you ever been driving and been thinking of something else? You suddenly get that unnerving feeling that you have not been consciously driving but you are still in one piece. How does this happen?

When our eyes are in peripheral we have access to our subconscious mind. If our conscious mind is busy it will take over. If you have driven that route before then all the details are stored in the subconscious and drives the car as if it is on autopilot. Scary or what?

When we are in peripheral vision we are also in a peak learning state. This is because we are accessing our all-powerful subconscious to learn for us.

The message here then is to be in peripheral vision as often as we can.

Relax

Sit back for a moment and spend five minutes relaxing. Focus on a point in front of you and just above your head. Now just relax your eyes and after a little while this should widen your vision. You can do this in your garden, a park or just look at a picture in a room. When you are completely relaxed just think of a problem or anything that is worrying you. If you keep in peripheral vision you will not be able to hold onto this thought. In my case the thought just seems to "fall through" and I am unable to catch it. This is the power of using your body to create and maintain a positive, relaxed state.

You can combine this with deep breathing and relaxing music if this works better.

It's time to feel good

I think that you will see that the more strategies and habits for feeling good we have at our disposal, the greater the chances are that we can feel good on an almost permanent basis.

We can all feel good if we are having a good day or even if our football team has won. The real challenge is for us to be able to call on our resources when we are tired, frustrated or in low mood. Here are a couple of ways to give yourself a boost when you most need it.

Whoosh

Sit comfortably or even lie down and just relax. Close your eyes and let the muscles around your eyes, your forehead, face and shoulders etc. relax. Now think of a time you were really, really happy. Bring that image up close to your face and turn up the colour of this special scene. Now step into your own body and see what you saw, feel what you felt and hear what you heard, etc. Really intensify that image so that you now have a big grin on your face. Turn up the volume and see if that helps.

Now push this image as far away in your mind as possible, so that it is a small dot in the bottom left hand corner of your "blank screen." Now say to yourself "Whoosh!" and bring the image in an instant back in full intensity back in front of your face. When you do this the image should almost knock your head backwards. Leave the image there and then shrink as before and then repeat.

Do that ten times and you should get a burst of positive feelings. This takes a little practice, but it can be done in a couple of minutes. You can do this on a train and people around you will just think you are having a pleasant nap.

The Circle of Confidence

Again close your eyes, and this time remember a time you felt really, really confident. Remember the confident strong, stance you had. Remember your steady breathing and your confident tone of voice. Now imagine that confidence is flowing from your solar plexus as a form of electric energy as you breathe out. Breathe in and out ten times and after each out breath feel this confident energy rising on this scale of one to ten.

After the tenth breath you should be tingling with positive energy. Now imagine that there is a white circle drawn in front of you and step into it. You can actually stand up and do this or just visualise this. Now that you are in the circle of confidence double this feeling again. You are now in a peak state!

Now spend as long as you can, imagining that this circle is around you, as you go about your day.

We have talked before about habits being very powerful. You may want to do one of these exercises at a set time each day. This way you get to <u>ensure</u> your positive state and remember that those around you might just catch your state too.

Things that make me feel happy

Another little thing we can do is to write out a list of ten things we can do that will improve our state. These are the little pleasures in life that can add up to a big difference. Again we have been conditioned by the media, advertising and society that we can only feel good if we have achieved something "significant". What a load of old baloney! If you want to be given a master class in happiness, then put this book down and go and watch a two year old playing with a cardboard box. There is great wisdom in watching children, as they can have fun anywhere. They do not feel any inhibitions. They are just happy because they are. They realise that this is their natural state.

P.S. When you have finished this please come back to me!

OK so here are my ten things that make me happy:

1.   Enjoying a joke with a friend.
2.   Watching *The Simpsons* or anything that makes me laugh.
3.   Listening to great music.
4.   Watching sports on TV.

5.   Reading a good book.
6.   Going for a walk along my local river.
7.   Exercising.
8.   Watching history programmes.
9.   Spending time with family and friends.
10.   Relaxing around nature.

So now it is your turn to think of ten things that you can do often that will make you feel good.

My top Ten Things

1.   ....
2.   ....
3.   ....
4.   ....
5.   ....
6.   ....
7.   ....
8.   ....
9.   ....
10.   ....

Don't think too hard and keep the list for reference. Perhaps you could just do one or two a day to bring a little variety into your routine. The message here as always is just to do what feels right for you.

Mind your language

Another area that has a huge impact on our state is our language. Both our internal and external language are vital in controlling how we feel.

Throughout history words have moved us to take action. It was once said that Winston Churchill sent the English language into battle. Generations have been inspired to do great things (and not so great of course) due to a speech.

Your inner voice

We are constantly talking to ourselves, if you hadn't noticed. From the moment we wake, until we drift off to sleep at night, we engage in this constant chatter. The problem is that often it is negative, and therefore we fill our minds with feelings of dread and overwhelm before we even brush our teeth. It is known that most heart attacks occur before 9am on a Monday, so this negativity is costing us dear.

Nature hates a vacuum, so we need to keep our self-talk positive so that we keep out the negative. It seems as if our "default position" is to be negative, so we must make a conscious effort to improve our thoughts. (I am English so apologies to those nations who are naturally more upbeat). Seriously, though, the chronic depression rates throughout the developed world should tell us that we all need to practice this. As with any skill, this gets easier and more natural with practice.

Words are powerful tools and we need to raise our awareness of how we use them so that they serve us and not hurt us. Remember that the bible says "something will master and something will serve." This is excellent advice and reminds us to be the master of our own thoughts and words.

How can we achieve this? By deliberately making your inner voice positive. When you wake up tomorrow just say to yourself "Thank you, thank you, thank you." Gratitude is such a positive emotion so thank your maker for a new day or just yourself for getting through the night.

Smile at yourself in the mirror and say "You look terrific!" This takes some imagination on my part but at least it makes me smile. Remember to affirm positively to yourself all day long –

"I like myself!"

"I can do it!"

"I feel terrific!"

"I am unstoppable!"

"I am a winner!"

Use these and add your own that have special meaning to you. This may seem difficult when you are having a lousy day, but repetition is the master skill. Just decide for tomorrow that whatever life throws at you, nothing is going to upset your new, positive peaceful mind. Just remember that we are only experiencing our perception of reality and nothing is 100% real. Let's create our own better reality that serves us well, and all those around us.

Watch your Mouth

Just as important as our inner voice are the words we speak. In England, during the Second World War, there were posters that said: "Careless words cost lives." This was meant to remind the civilian population that there could be enemy spies lurking around every street corner.

This still applies to us all today. We may not be in a military war but we should all stand guard at the door of our minds. Our subconscious is silently recording everything we say and using this as evidence against us. The habit of negative talk can literally shorten our lives.

Advertisers have known for decades how words can affect our state and therefore motivate us to buy. They do this by endless repetition or brand positioning as the marketers call it. If you hear the words "Just do it" what brand springs to your mind? I still remember the song from an advert in the 1970s that started "I'd like to teach the world to sing in perfect harmony." I still associate it in my mind with a certain popular soft drink!

The point here is that advertisers can imprint their message on us by constant exposure from the media. Similarly we are constantly advertising to ourselves about how we see ourselves, and our place in the world, through our words.

Observation is the key here, so just for a day, listen to the words you say to yourself and also to others.

This is an area where a negative upbringing can have a seriously damaging effect on a person. Emotional abuse can have as bad an effect on someone as physical abuse. This means that we have to be sensitive both of our words to ourselves and others. The expression about sticks and stones is easy to say but we have all said something in the heat of the moment that we just cannot take back. The good news is that we can transform our relationship with ourselves, and others, by only using positive language. The old adage that "if you can't think of something good to say about someone then say nothing" is a pretty good one to live by.

Do you think that people who constantly bad mouth people are happy? We have already talked about the law of attraction so what do you think we attract if we are negative about someone else? More negativity of course. Tell me something – do you think your life would be better with more negativity? If you have answered yes then why you are reading this book is a mystery. The point is that we damage ourselves if we put down ourselves or others. There is no place for this if we want to enjoy and build a happy, healthy personality. This is something I have to keep working on but we are all works in progress. Progress is of course the key. We must just keep heading in the right direction – the direction of happiness.

Change your words, change your future

After understanding this, I realised that a lot of my phrases and words were disempowering and just set me up for a fall. Phrases like –

"Why does this always happen to me?"

"I could never do that."

"I am totally exhausted."

"I am furious."

"You have really p****d me off."

I have tried, through practice to change these to –

"What can I learn from this?"

"Of course you can do it."

"I am getting out of state."

"I need to recharge myself."

"I am allowing myself to get annoyed."

Hopefully you can see that the second group of phrases lessen the emotional intensity of the moment. They also allow me to take responsibility for my state and some also give a solution to the situation. This is the difference of reacting to life and responding in an appropriate way. The more control we have over our emotions the better our lives will be. We cannot always control what others say or do but only our own responses.

This is about replacing disempowering words and phrases and replacing them with empowering ones.

That said, list a few of these phrases below that you know you need to replace –

Old Phrases

....

....

....

....

....

And replace them with your own new empowering ones –

<u>New Phrases</u>

....

....

....

....

....

This process is about raising our awareness as to what does not serve us and letting these things go and bringing into our lives things that do.

The power of questions

A large part of our language is in the form of questions. Our questions decide what we focus on, either positive or negative. For example if someone keeps looking at themselves in a mirror and asks "Why can't I lose any weight?" what are they focussing on? Obviously the fact that they cannot lose weight which is a negative thought. This is causing them to focus on the problem and not the solution. Furthermore the mind of this person will come up with an appropriately unhelpful answer, such as "because you are stupid and lazy." Not good.

A better question would be "How can I lose this weight?" This simple change in words focusses the person's mind on to positive, constructive answers and solutions. "Why" questions tend to focus us on excuses, (I must be big boned) whilst "how" questions focus towards solutions (I could go for a walk after dinner every night). As long as we are focused on solutions and not just excuses, then there is hope of progress. Where attention goes, energy flows. Just writing this stuff is putting me in a better mood. I hope the same is true of you as you read it.

Many of the world's greatest achievements have come after someone dared to ask the question "how?" How can we put a man on the moon? How can man fly like the birds? How can man communicate without wires? How can women get the vote?

If we keep asking good questions, then eventually we will get a good answer. Again it is about trusting that the little genius that resides in us all will appear when we most need him or her.

Life is like an old long playing record. At first the needle turns slowly around the edge and life moves at a slow pace. As we get older the needle speeds up as we get closer to the end. Of course at the end of the record there is just a hole that we will all fall into. Where that hole leads to is a separate question.

What this means is that we must seize the day and start implementing change as soon as possible. Little and often is the motto here.

Symbols and metaphors

Symbols can have a powerful effect on our state. Most people would look at their national flag with a sense of pride. Indeed, a flag is symbolic of what that country represents in terms of its values etc. It is a great insult to see your own flag being burnt in the streets by another people. If you are a Christian then a simple cross can move you inside. Yet if they saw a picture of a burning cross the same person might recoil in disgust.

Countries, organisations, political parties and companies take great care with their symbols, as they are all aware of the power they can have on us. Think of all the symbols that mean a lot to you. It could be that of your favourite sports team, food, political party or a symbol of your spiritual beliefs. Symbols connect with our subconscious mind which is why we have strong feelings towards them. Photographs are also very powerful as they are symbols or representations of those we love. Make sure that your important symbols are placed where you can see them each day. These little details all add up to greatly improve our mood and therefore our effectiveness.

Metaphors are expressions we use to liken something to something else. For example if I said that "The weight of the world is on my shoulders" then you would know that I was feeling under pressure. If I said "I feel like I am skipping on air" then you would know that I was in an energised state.

Again this is an opportunity to raise your awareness as to which metaphors are helping you and which are not. Observation without any judgement on yourself is the key here. We are breaking old habits which have run silent and deep. So deep that we are oblivious to them unless we take special notice of them.

Winston Churchill once said that an iron curtain had descended across Europe. He was describing how Europe had been divided by Communism, and it was a great metaphor to describe decades of oppression. Indeed, when Communism fell we can all remember pictures of people breaking up the Berlin Wall. They could easily have just walked through the open gates to the west, but they wanted to destroy what they viewed as the symbol of their oppression: the wall.

Putting it all together

This subject of our state is a huge topic and, as you can now see, there are multiple factors that determine how we feel. The good news here is that, conversely, there are many simple but effective things we can do to ensure our state. We do not need to be a victim of circumstances in that we can now largely shape how we experience them. We have the tools.

Firstly, remember that our minds act as filters deleting, distorting and generalising our experiences to create our perception of reality. This explains why two people could have a totally different point of view. They are both right and wrong at the same time. Something to think about.

Secondly, our physiology has a massive impact on our states. Indeed we do our states through our body movements. We need to realise this and breathe deeply, keep in peripheral vision, stand tall and smile. We can also break our less resourceful states in an instant with our bodies.

Lastly, we must use the power of our language to achieve and maintain a positive state. Words are powerful tools, so choose your tools wisely to get the job done. The job in question is your ongoing contentment and growth.

Remember also the power of asking empowering questions, as these focus our minds on solutions and new possibilities. Watch out that you are also using positive metaphors and surround yourself with the symbols that are special to you.

I am sure you found this subject interesting. What could be more interesting than learning how to make yourself happy in an instant? This is all about taking responsibility for our state. It is about being in charge. We need to take a proactive approach to our happiness. Managing and controlling our state is a great way to do this.

ACTION POINTS

- Realise that nothing you experience is 100% real. Use this to lessen the intensity of your bad experiences.

- Use your body to keep yourself in a happy, resourceful state.

- Think of as many ways as possible for you to quickly feel good. Write them down.

- Mind your language. You may want to refer to a dictionary or thesaurus and find new, more empowering words to use from now on.

- Use the whoosh technique to kick start yourself into a good mood.

- Review your use of questions, symbols and metaphors. Respect their power to shift your state.

- Remember that all these little changes really add up to make a big difference in your life.

I trust that you really get the importance of all this. Most importantly I hope you are waking up to the enormous power you have inside you that is just waiting to be put to use. Our only question now should be: What are we going to do with all this power?

In the next chapter we are going to explore an area that is vital to our personal growth and development. It is something you are doing by reading this book and it is my belief that in order to get the most out of life, we must make a firm commitment to...

CHAPTER 6

EDUCATE

"In times of change, learners inherit the earth, while the learned find themselves beautifully equipped to deal with a world that no longer exists." – Eric Hoffer.

I am sure by now that you are enjoying this process. This next part of our journey together is all about the joy of learning. I say joy because nothing makes us feel more alive than when we are learning and growing. It is said that six out of ten adults never read an educational book after they leave full time education. This is certainly not for us.

I believe this negative association with learning is the result of our archaic educational system. I say this with confidence because psychologists have known since the 1960s that the way we teach in our schools does not work.

In experiments done at this time it was shown that passive learning, where you are expected to absorb information whilst you sit, is the least effective way to learn. The more active the student is in the learning process, say through an activity or an experiment, the quicker he or she learns. This is why I have designed this book so that you not only read the information, but you reinforce the learning through practical activities.

As well as trying to passively learn things, even worse is that we are told what it is we will learn. By the time we are fourteen most of the students begin to question what practical use is of what they are learning. I don't know about you but I have never had the need to make copper sulphate, use trigonometry or dissect a frog in the thirty years that I have left the education system.

Contrast that with adults who attend educational classes because they want to be there. I am sure the motivation to learn is much higher as a result and, of course, they are paying for it. Here are the results of that earlier experiment:-

Cone of Learning

After 2 weeks we tend to remember		Nature of Involvement
90% of what we say and do	Doing the Real Thing	Active
	Simulating the Real Experience	
	Doing a Dramatic Presentation	
70% of what we say	Giving a Talk	
	Participating in a Discussion	
50% of what we hear and see	Seeing it Done on Location	Passive
	Watching a Demonstration	
	Looking at an Exhibit Watching a Demonstration	
	Watching a Movie	
30% of what we see	Looking at Pictures	
20% of what we hear	Hearing Words	
10% of what we read	Reading	

This diagram demonstrates that we learn best by doing. First we must learn and then put it into use. Knowledge without action is useless. We only know something if we practice it. The word educate comes from the Latin verb meaning to take out or draw out. This means that education is not really about absorbing information but drawing out of us what is already there, and finding new distinctions as a result.

Lao Tzu once said "Knowing others is intelligence; knowing yourself is true wisdom. Mastering others is strength; mastering yourself is true power." This process of learning is as much about discovering what is inside ourselves as it is about learning new information.

Personal growth is about stretching ourselves and moulding ourselves for a brighter future. It is exciting and, above all, it should be fun. Again I will refer to young children here. Children have an insatiable appetite for learning. Indeed the period from birth until seven years old is known as the quantum learning period. It is time that we reconnected with the child within and rediscover the joy that comes from learning.

Another problem that we have with education is that it is a slow, ongoing process. We live in an age of instant gratification – and soon that will not be fast enough! Statistics show that we will browse a web page for an average of seven seconds before clicking away. We will look at the front cover of a book for six seconds and the back cover for nine seconds before we decide whether to buy it or not. We are easily bored and seventy per cent of the time we watch television we are channel hopping.

Malcolm Gladwell states, in his book *Outliers*, that it takes someone ten thousand hours to master any subject. That is roughly five years of working forty hours a week at it. This is what it takes to master any field. Success is not an overnight thing. The five years is going to pass anyway so we might as well learn something along the way.

What should I learn?

This is really a personal choice but I concentrate on learning anything that will help me achieve my goals. Let's review those areas again.

Health

This is one of the most important areas you can study. With the internet there is of course more information available than ever before. The fact that my local library is filled with health books shows there is a real interest in this subject. I heard a horrible statistic the other day that stated the average person will soon expend only 25% more energy than if they had stayed in bed all day. Our sedentary lives and our diets of processed food means that we are slowly killing ourselves. We are digging our graves with our teeth.

The great news here is that science has proved that we can reverse a lot of this damage by simply changing our habits. The pay offs for focusing your efforts in this area are greater energy, being your ideal weight, greater life expectancy and getting the best out of life.

Relationships

The fact that you are caring for a loved one shows me that you are a role model in this area. Indeed one of the great pluses of caring is a deep, loving connection with those closest to you. Family is such an important unit and studies have again shown repeatedly that we live longer and happier lives in a loving environment.

With regard to intimate relationships, I was fascinated when I explored the subject of male and female energy. You have probably heard of Yin (female) and Yang (male) energy in spirituality. We have both, regardless of our gender, although one is usually much stronger than the other. Masculine energy tends to be focused on a result and is usually seen as being assertive. It is also protective towards the feminine. This energy is typified by the alpha male go-getter type.

Feminine energy is typified as a sort of radiance. It is not focused, but radiates outwards in all directions. Think of a woman playing with her baby and you will sense the type of harmonious, loving energy that exudes from the mother. Both energies are attracted to each other. Even in same sex relationships one partner will show feminine energy whilst the other exudes masculine energy. I realised after learning this, that relationships are a fascinating dance between these two energies. Indeed one cannot thrive without the other.

Money

This is an area that affects all the others, whether we like it or not. Again money is just an energy that is designed to flow. Our educational system again fails to teach us anything about this subject. We tend to pick up the beliefs and attitudes of our parents to guide us through life. If you repeatedly heard "Money doesn't grow on trees" then often we can go through life with a scarcity mentality.

The fact is that the universe is an abundant place and it is expanding all the time. In his book *The Science of Getting Rich*, Wallace D. Wattles stated the following –

"It requires power to think health when surrounded by the appearance of disease, or to think riches when in the midst of the appearances of poverty. But, he who acquires this power becomes a mastermind. He can conquer fate; he can have what he wants."

Very true. It takes a lot of belief to think of abundance when you are in a state of scarcity. However, abundance is the natural state of the universe. We have been fooled by the media and society to be both not content with and to settle for what we currently have. We should be grateful for what we have whilst we pursue all that we want. I would recommend a book by T. Harv. Ecker called "The Millionaire Mind". It gives a great insight into the mind-set of the wealthy. Remember that success all happens in the mind.

Lifestyle

Another great area to study is the art of living well. We have already talked about so many little things that we can do on a daily basis, which make life just that little bit better. This is about compounding these little rituals and gaining momentum in our lives. I cannot remind you too often that happiness equals progress. Jim Rohn wrote a book and audio series called "The art of exceptional Living". Jim explained that a great life is not always about doing great things. It is about doing the simple things in life exceptionally well. I think that this is a great insight.

If we can just make small and frequent improvements in all that we do then this compounds into an enjoyable life.

If we have little money we can live with elegant simplicity. Really enjoy that walk in the park, place a simple bunch of flowers in our home and enjoy our friends and family to the fullest. Study the art of happiness and you will not be disappointed.

<u>Goals</u>

More than anything else we have discussed, goals give us direction and a stronger sense of purpose. They tell us how we will spend our time. They also tell us what we need to learn. In the first chapter on mentors we covered the fact that someone else has often achieved what we want to be, do or have.

Luckily a lot of successful people have put their stories into books. There we can learn their triumphs, their struggles, their disasters and their ultimate victory. You will find that most of these special people are in reality, ordinary people just like you and me. What is extraordinary about them is that they all refused to settle for anything less than their dreams. In life we get what we settle for.

Write out some goals and refer to them often. If you were to write out ten goals and put the paper in a drawer; a year later you would be amazed that you had accomplished most of them. Goals really concentrate the mind and remember to bring in emotional visualisation to allow the power of your subconscious to do its magic. What if I don't hit my goals? Well perhaps you were not meant to but keep persevering. God's delays are not God's denials. Perhaps you will receive an even greater blessing as a result. We cannot lose if we just take action and trust in our own abilities. Every failure has within it a nugget of wisdom that is priceless if we learn from it.

Contribution

The more we learn the more we can contribute to others. It is that simple. Often we can contribute to others by being a role model. Having a deep desire to learn often comes from our fundamental need to contribute. The attitude you have when you are eager to learn will affect others around you. Sharing what you know with others is real generosity.

Teaching others is also a great way to learn at a deeper level. The teacher always receives the best lesson. Writing this book is stretching me and forcing me to learn this stuff at a higher level. I am grateful for that. Another great way to teach is through stories. Jesus was the master story teller and taught Christian principles through them. All I can remember of my bible classes were the famous stories of Herod, the Good Samaritan and Samson to name but a few.

Learning how to contribute more to our loved ones, our friends and society gives a great sense of well-being, pride and contentment.

Purpose

This is the reason that you were uniquely put on the planet. Your purpose will also be your passion. It is what defines you as a human being. It does not have to be grandiose to be important, and it can change as your life changes. If your purpose is to be a great carer then is that sufficient? Of course. Caring for someone else is one of the most meaningful ways to live your purpose. It may not always be glamorous but it can lead to a deep sense of fulfilment and peace of mind. Now that is real success.

Personal Growth

Nothing, of course, helps with our growth as much as learning. Every time we learn something we are developing as individuals. Our knowledge is compounding and we begin to view life differently. This is a lifelong process and this book is just another step in this exciting journey.

Learning keeps us focused on solutions and not on problems. It is not what we get that is valuable but who we become. Who knows what you can become as our potential is unlimited. Learners are happier, have more energy and keep themselves young at heart. We can never be bored if we develop a healthy curiosity. Learning gives us momentum and direction. There is a saying to do with exercise; "use it or lose it." The same is true of our mental muscles; we must use what we have or our mind can go into decline. Research has repeatedly shown that we can maintain and protect our minds by regularly challenging them.

Mind-set

We cannot do anything until we first think about it. Our thoughts are affected by many factors, as we have covered earlier. Therefore the study of how and why we think is one of the best ways you can spend your time. If we can change the quality of our thinking, we can change our results and ultimately our lives.

Correct thinking positively affects every area of our lives, from our health to our relationships. Napoleon Hill said "We become what we think about." This is very true. This is why positive people live positive, healthy, productive lives and negative people attract the exact opposite into their lives. To paraphrase the bible; the more you give thanks, the more you will have to be grateful for.

This is the law of attraction at work. I always seem to get more things to moan about as a result of moaning. I am sure you have experienced this too. This is why a state of gratitude is so important. Throughout human history man has been fascinated by this subject of how we think, and we will cover this in much greater detail later.

But I don't have the time

I realise that your plate is pretty full right now. The demands on your day must seem overwhelming at times. If our ultimate resource is our resourcefulness, then we have to be creative in how we use our time. Audio learning, as we have discussed, is a great way to learn whilst we are driving, doing house work and even exercising.

If someone read for one hour a day, they would read approximately one book a week. That is around fifty books a year. In ten years they would have read five hundred books! Imagine what they could do with their knowledge. Imagine their confidence.

I understand the average person watches around four hours of TV a day. If they just used one of those hours to read then they could, over time, transform themselves. Even if you are a slow reader you can pick up an enormous amount of information with only thirty minutes study a day. As always just start where you can and build this into an enjoyable hobby. We live in the information age where knowledge is power. The days of someone doing the same job for forty years and then retiring on a nice, safe company pension have gone. Go and read the quote at the start of the chapter again. It is no good nowadays to rely on previous qualifications, as the world is moving too quickly. If we are not moving forwards then we are moving backwards. Put yourself on the side of the angels and get learning.

The shop of life

Once again I am indebted to the late Jim Rohn here. I am never afraid to use someone else's work because I would never have thought of it myself! Jim once said that imagine you entered the shop of life. In this shop there is everything that life has to offer, both good and bad. You notice that everything you don't want is close to hand and easy to grab. You notice, however, that everything that you want from life is out of reach. Wisdom, health, abundance and friendship are all on the very top shelf of the shop.

The lesson here is that there is only one way to reach the good things in life. You have to first stand on all the good books that you have read. Now it is easy to have all those good things. I thought that was such a great analogy that I had to share it with you. We had better pick up the books.

Body language

As over half of our communication is body language, this is a useful area to study. Subconsciously we are already experts, as we can usually tell the slightest change in mood in those around us. Imagine a scene where you walked into a bar or social gathering, and the volume was turned down. I am sure you could tell if people were at ease with each other or not. Usually when two or more people are in harmony with each other their body language will match. They will even take sips from their glasses at the same time. If suddenly there was a disagreement, it would be obvious because suddenly there would be a mismatch in their body language.

The idea of matching and mirroring has been around for a while and you have probably heard of it. Matching is where if you raise your right hand I raise my right hand. Mirroring is when you raise your right hand I raise my left hand to mirror you.

We tend to like people who are similar to us, so if we subtlety adopt the other person's body language then we can build an effective rapport. The technique is to notice how the other person sits and match if they sit back or lean forward. When they talk breathe out to match their breathing. If they use their arms a lot then gesticulate when you reply.

The best way to impress someone is to be impressed by them. The best way to do this is by giving them the gift of attention. Keep eye contact with the person as they speak, lean slightly forward and nod to indicate agreement. If you feel uncomfortable with too much eye contact, then look at the general area of the face and upper torso. This way you don't have to say much and the other person will enjoy your company. I am sure you have had this experience.

If you want to persuade someone then here is a simple technique. If you want to emphasise that you possess a certain quality (hard-working, loyal, confident, etc.) then you need to use your body language and well as your words. In a job interview, for example, every time you say that you are hard-working, touch your upper chest area with your finger tips of one or both hands. This action anchors the idea of you being hard-working into the subconscious mind of the interviewer. They will not notice as long as it is not overdone and this is a powerful way to persuade. You can just touch your tie or your necklace every time you want to emphasise one of your qualities.

Public speaking

One of the best things I have ever done is to take a course in public speaking. In America it is people's number one fear before even death. In the UK only the fear of spiders is higher! This just shows that I can't make these facts up. Psychologists state, that if you can speak well in public, then people will often credit you with an intelligence that you do not necessarily possess. Let's keep that one to ourselves, eh? Here are a few tips on how to be more effective in this area.

Eye contact

You know how the nerves kick in when you are faced with an audience. Firstly, try to keep your eyes relaxed and stay in peripheral vision. I used to look above the heads of everyone to avoid eye contact with anyone. The problem with that is that you lose any engagement. Instead look randomly at people as if you are talking directly to that one person. Hold eye contact for a few seconds and then pick someone else out to talk to. This helps you to engage much better with your audience.

Stance

It is easy to go into a defensive type stance, with your arms crossed or hands in your pockets. Instead stand with your feet a little less than shoulder width apart and pointing in front towards the group. This makes you look taller and more confident. Then imagine there is a string coming out of the top of your head. This string is pulling you gently upright so that your back is straight.

Next place your hands together at just above belt level. I place one hand above the other with palms facing up to the ceiling. The important thing is not to cross your arms. From this position use your hands freely to emphasise what you are saying but always bring them back to this neutral position.

Breathing

When we are nervous our breathing is fast and shallow. This is not good for talking in public, so we need to deal with it. Before you speak you can do ten breaths in and out to the count of ten to get your breathing under control. The important thing to realise is that we breathe out when we speak. This sounds obvious but it is easy to forget when under pressure.

When you speak, speak slowly. This will help to control your breathing. Also pause often. This will give your audience time to digest what you are saying and give you time to remember what you were going to say next! Walking around also keeps the attention of people and can help you control your breathing.

Be yourself

As a student of public speaking I would try to copy the best. It is good to see how successful people perform and to incorporate it into your speaking. People though, want to hear you speak and not just another clone. You don't have to be word perfect. People are not so concerned in hearing a sterile, perfect, polished performance but want to hear what you believe in. We have already mentioned that people will like you if they feel similar to you. The clue here then is to be similar and not special. Keep your focus on your audience and let your words serve them.

Every speaker's greatest fear is to dry up and forget what you are going to say. A great piece of advice I heard was that you would meet a friend and chat away for a good hour or two without any notes! You do not script out your conversations or try to memorise them in advance. Just have a clear idea of the main areas you want to cover and you will be fine. You might just enjoy yourself and this is one of the best ways to build your self-esteem and confidence.

Your success rules

Success does not happen by accident; it leaves clues. A valuable exercise is to review on paper the last twelve months or so. Start with all the things you have accomplished whether you set out to do them or not. Allow yourself to feel good as you will probably surprise yourself when you look back at all you did.

Now note down everything you failed to do or achieve in the same period. This is not so pleasant but no one achieves everything they want to. Note down the reasons that you achieved your goals. Was it good time management? Did you make them a priority? Did you approach the task with certainty? Did you ask the right person for advice? Write as many reasons as you can think.

These reasons will be your personal rules for success. Now if you think about the goals you didn't achieve, the chances are that you broke these success rules. Why not copy these out onto 5 x 3 inch card and carry them round with you? They will be there to remind you what works for you. They are your golden rules and will ensure your consistency from now on.

I forgive you

Most personal development books cover the importance of forgiveness. The idea is that, in order for us to move on with our lives, we must forgive everyone that has ever hurt us.

This sounds logical, in that by forgiving, we are dropping our emotional baggage. This baggage weighs us down and slows our progress to true happiness. However, in spite of intellectually grasping this, I still found it hard to let go of my anger and resentment to people who I felt had wronged me in some way. I had this underlying feeling that if I forgave someone, that I was somehow "letting them off the hook." I wanted them punished. This is, of course, the opposite of forgiveness and caused me much emotional conflict. I was taking one step forward and then one back as my anger dissipated and then reappeared.

The answer came recently in the form of an email from Dr Robert Anthony. After reading this article by him on forgiveness, a sentence popped into my head which instantly changed my life. It might well change yours if you truly grasp its power. The sentence is simply this:

Nothing happens To me, everything happens FOR me. Read that again slowly as it could change your thinking forever!

This means that no one is rude or nasty to us, they are rude or nasty for us. They have been sent to teach us a lesson. They have been sent to help us. We only have to observe and find the valuable lesson. This thought leads to gratitude. If we are grateful then we do not need to forgive. There is literally nothing to forgive. Do you realise what power you now have? If everything happens for your benefit then anger, frustration and depression just disappear from your life.

If we forgive someone then we hold something over them. This thought is coming from our ego (subconscious) which likes to keep us trapped in negativity. The thought of being happy scares our ego, as this equals change. It wants us to play the victim by remaining angry and even depressed because of something that happened twenty years ago. I cover negativity in its many guises in much greater detail in the next chapter.

Never seek revenge. The universe hates imbalance and it will punish the person as it sees fit. It is none of your business. If the universe does not punish them then it was just meant to be. We just need to focus on being grateful for the lesson. Sometimes I learn it and sometimes I don't. I am getting better as this is a skill that needs constant practice to master.

We can now look back at our life and let go of any resentment we have to others. I am truly grateful to Dr Anthony for giving me this priceless gift. That gift is a life that has replaced anger with gratitude. I never need to play the victim again.

I included this into this chapter on learning for a reason. If we want to discover a nugget of gold we have to shift tonnes of dirt. I have read countless books and articles before I found this nugget of wisdom. I can tell you that it was well worth all the effort. It's time to crack open the books.

Conclusion

All leaders are readers. We have seen that a daily small discipline like reading thirty minutes a day, can have a dramatic compounding effect on our knowledge. We can transform our skill sets and our whole perspective on life. We can discover new talents and abilities that have lain dormant within us. It is time to release the little wizard within you.

The idea that learning is boring often comes from bad memories of school. Unlike at school, teacher is not standing over you telling you what you will learn. Be like a child in a sweet shop and explore all the possibilities. Find a learning style you enjoy or a combination. Some days I don't want to read so I just listen to a CD or sit down and watch a DVD or online video. Experiment and have fun.

Most people are like pavlovian dogs just accepting whatever rubbish the TV producers deem fit to serve up. We all need to relax with our favourite show but don't let the TV rule your life. Sorry if I sound like I am preaching but I will cover later the damage TV does to people. Your life is too precious not to be put to better use.

ACTION POINTS

- Review your daily schedule and see if you could free up any time to learn.
- Be creative. Could you use that commute or drive to the shops better by listening to something educational? How about the same idea when you walk the dog?
- Remember that it can take just thirty minutes a day to begin a new life of learning.
- What do you want to learn? Reviewing your goals is a great place to start.
- Have you ever thought to yourself "I wonder if I could do that?" Perhaps you can.
- Imagine all the things you could be, do and have with what you will learn.
- Realise that in five years we will all be five years older. We might as well be five years smarter as well.
- Above all learn at the pace that is right for you. There is no rush. You are on the right path. Just put one foot in front of the other and gradually your whole life will change.

The next chapter is possibly the most important in this entire book. If we do this right we can transform our entire destiny and of those around us. Above all else we must master the ability to…

CHAPTER 7

THINK

"The world as we have created it is a process of our thinking. It cannot be changed without changing our thinking." – Albert Einstein

Human beings have been given the remarkable ability to think. Compared with any other species we are all geniuses. This has lead the human race to reign supreme over all other life forms. This great gift is the human brain. It is the most complex, brilliant creation in nature.

Unfortunately for us, this incredibly powerful tool that sits between our ears, does not come with an instruction manual. The fact is we continue to pollute the earth and continue to destroy countless species of life every year. This tells us that we often do not use our cognitive powers wisely. At least two billion people live on less than two US dollars a day. This is in spite of there being more money in the world than ever before. Millions of people die each year from easily treatable diseases, as well as wars and genocide.

The positive side to this incredible ability to think, is that we have also used our minds constructively to create incredible advances in technology, science, medicine and in numerous other areas. This speed of progress is advancing exponentially. Indeed it is only ten years ago that you had to dial up for an internet connection; and how did anyone live without a smart phone?

Although it seems like we have been given these awesome mental powers, we have received little guidance on how to think. The school system tends to focus us on what to think. This is really an extraordinary oversight and urgently needs attention if we are to build a fairer and more peaceful world. This requires a raising of the collective consciousness of everyone on the planet. Now that is a tall order! What we can do is to focus on changing and improving our own thoughts a little bit each day.

The industrialist Henry Ford once stated; "Thinking is the hardest work there is, which is probably the reason so few engage in it." The fact is that going inside your own mind and analysing your thoughts can be quite scary. This is a process of observing your thoughts but not judging them. Judgement leads to negative self-talk which is not helpful. We are after the courage to discover why we think the way we do. Remember that Lao-Tzu said that to know oneself is true wisdom.

We are seeking wisdom; the wisdom that is inside all of us.

Thoughts are energy

Science has proved beyond doubt that everything is energy. Everything that is formed was once formless. Every particle was formed from waves of energy. This means that our thoughts are energy. This is important for us to know as this has everything to do with our own happiness.

Positive thoughts are a form of positive energy which, in turn, attracts more positive energy. This explains why optimists live longer than pessimists. This is why it is imperative that we keep our thoughts predominantly positive. We attract into our lives what we think about; good or bad. This is why we must search for the positive meaning in every problem and set back, however difficult that may be. As we can only hold one conscious thought in our heads, then the key is to keep those thoughts positive.

I will be happy when...

I am sure you have heard the Beach Boys song called "Good Vibrations." When we think, we are producing vibrational energy. All energy vibrates and attracts other energy with a similar vibration. I know this all sounds a bit "new age" but I promise I have not been smoking anything that I shouldn't. This is science. Don't ask me how this works. All we need to know is that it works and to use this knowledge to our advantage.

In order to be happy in the future, we must be happy now. The future never arrives anyway. All we have is a series of "now" moments in our lives. We have been conditioned to believe that we will be happy when...

I get married.

I get divorced.

I lose this weight.

I get the new house.

I have kids.

The kids leave the house. Etc., etc.

Remember that wherever you go, there you are. We cannot delay our happiness. Happiness has to be now or it is never. Happiness cannot be dependent on any future event. What if this never happens? Even if this does happen to us we tend to quickly revert back to our usual level of happiness. I am sure you have experienced this many times in the past. Happiness is often found in the journey and not in the destination. It is our western culture that dictates that our happiness must depend on a certain set of circumstances. This just leads to frustration and disappointment if things do not work out the way we wanted. We must be happy with what we have whilst we pursue all that we want. We do not need to wait. Indeed we must not wait. To quote Wayne Dyer: There is no way to happiness, happiness is the way.

Avoid Materialism

There was a recent study done to discover if there is a relationship between materialism and self-esteem. They found that materialism actually increases low self-esteem. The researchers at the University of Illinois found that as an individual's self-esteem increases, their interest in materialism decreases. The study focused on children and adolescents. This is what the researchers had to say on this subject –

"By the time children reach early adolescence and experience a decline in self-esteem, the stage is set for the use of material possessions as a coping strategy for feelings of low self-worth. The paradox is that consumerism is good for the economy in the short term, but bad for the individual in the long run, especially young people. Most of us want more income so that we can consume more stuff. However, several separate studies show as societies become richer, they do not become happier. Statistically people have more material possessions and money than fifty years ago, but they are actually less happy. In fact, the wealthiest countries have more depression, alcoholism and more crime than they did fifty years ago and yet we have more material goods to purchase than ever before. This paradox is true of Britain, The United States, Australia, Europe and Japan.

The real reason people want whatever is "hot" or "in style" is because they believe it will contribute to their happiness and satisfaction in life. Research shows time and time again that this very belief is false."

The answer is to <u>choose to be happy now</u>. That way we can cut out the credit card bill. Think about the last time you were truly happy. I am guessing that it had a fairly simple and non- commercial nature to it. The simple things really do make us happy, despite what all those adverts say.

Where are my keys?

Imagine if you were leaving your home and your neighbour was on his knees, seemingly looking for something. Naturally you would ask her what she was looking for and she replies that she has lost her keys. Now being a good neighbour you start to help her look.

After a few minutes you ask her where exactly she lost her keys. With a pleasant smile on her face, she informs you that she dropped them in the kitchen. At this point you just might ask her what you are both doing on your knees on her drive! This seemingly silly story has an important message: are we all looking for happiness in the wrong place? If we are then it is not surprising that so many people are unhappy. Something to think about.

Stay Focused

I have just been watching a recording of a very successful businessman speaking at an event in London. I always try to learn something when someone speaks. It is usually only a matter of time before you learn something of value. Anyway, he gave this piece of advice which happens to hold great wisdom for us. His advice was simply; "Focus on what you want." Simple but incredibly profound. I have written those words on a piece of paper and stuck it on my refrigerator door.

We should always be willing to learn from those around us and I am grateful for the advice. Most of the time we are focusing on what we don't want which is, of course attracting more of what we don't want into our lives. We use the law of attraction against us. By focusing on what we want we are using this law very much to our advantage. We need, like the mountain climber, to keep our eyes and minds focused on the summit.

Be quiet

We talk to ourselves twenty-four hours a day. Often it seems nearly impossible to shut up our thoughts. A useful technique is to be able to interrupt our thoughts and bring in "no mind." This is where you literally think of nothing. This may sound easy, but try doing it right now and see how you get on. The first time I did this it was less than five seconds before the next annoying thought popped into my mind.

The next time you are alone, sit or lie down and close your eyes. Turn off all noises or distractions for a few moments. Close your eyes and relax. Then say to yourself something like; "What am I going to think about next?" Your mind should clear for a few seconds. The first few times you do this, you will do well to keep a thought out for more than ten seconds. Don't worry but congratulate yourself that for those few seconds at least, you were in charge of your mind. This is very soothing and helps to "reset" the mind. The question interrupts the constant chatter that continuously plagues us all. If you practice, you can soon get up to a minute, which is fine. This is another simple form of meditation. Buddhist monks can meditate for hours on end every day. They are seeking enlightenment, which is a state of total bliss where you realise that you do not need anything. Indeed The Buddha said "All desire creates suffering." Contrast that to our consumer driven society.

I do not believe that any one philosophy has all the answers, but we need to be flexible in our thinking, and be open to using anything that can serve us. We do not need or have the time to meditate three hours a day. Just bring in no mind for a minute or so a few times a day and you will feel the difference. Again it says in the bible that "something will master and something will serve." It is time we took back control of our minds one little step at a time. The secret is to not try to bring in no mind but rather just to relax. Say the question and let your mind clear. I can do this walking down the street, exercising and listening to music. This is just another tool in our tool box that we can use. We discussed earlier there are plenty of music tracks, DVDs, CDs, books that you can meditate to if you want to explore this area further. You are not wasting your time by learning to strengthen your mind and body. It beats watching TV!

Slow down

Common thinking has it that we have to be doing something every moment of the day. We spend our days rushing around trying to cram more and more into our busy lives. This is not great for our health and happiness. Just because someone is busy, it does not mean they are being productive. Busyness can be a form of laziness. Remember what Henry Ford said about thinking being the hardest work there is. Most people would rather be busy than spend time on the discipline of controlling their minds. Think about this: There is no rushing in nature but everything always gets done.

We need to be focused but not rushing. If we rush we often spend half our time undoing our mistakes. If someone comes to my home to fix something, I like to slow them down. I give them a coffee, biscuits and have a little chat with them. I want them to spend those few extra minutes to do a good job. I do not want them to rush and do a sloppy job. We must be the same and work and live at a slower, more methodical pace. Keeping our minds relaxed actually gives us more energy to be more effective in our daily lives.

Be...Do...Have

Everything that man has created started as a thought in someone's mind. The formless thought became the formed object. Look around at everything you own as they all started as just an idea. This is the power of thought.

One of the problems with New Year resolutions is that the person focuses on the doing i.e. exercising or saving. If we want lasting change we must focus on the being. How can we change who we are? By changing our thoughts. This entire book is about changing our thinking so that it consistently empowers and serves us. Yes we all have bad days, but the trick is to gain something positive from it. A good question to ask ourselves is how can this serve me? There is always value to any situation. Sometimes it takes some creativity though!

If we focus on how we think then our actions in turn change, which leads to a better result or outcome. In other words, to be healthy, we have to think like a healthy person and adopt their attitudes, values and beliefs. The easiest way to do this is by learning from them. Observation here is important as success leaves clues. We must become a good observer of the people who do and have what we desire.

Acceptance is the key

If we want to experience ongoing contentment and peace of mind, we have to accept what is. Non acceptance leads to anger and frustration, which is the opposite of what we want. We have to accept what is because we have to accept reality. We may not like a situation and we can do our best to change it. However, we must accept that we are where we are at any given moment in time.

To fight against reality is madness and will just leave us bitter and exhausted. We must accept we are where we are and deal with it in the present moment. Acceptance gives us the ability to deal with a crisis in a calmer manner. I say calmer depending on the situation of course.

As well as accepting our circumstances, we have to accept and love ourselves, in spite of our faults and actions. We all make mistakes, so just accept it and move on. You are probably thinking that this is not possible but it is the only way we can change our future. There is true peace in acceptance.

Be Present

Next we must learn to become predominantly present. Most of our time our ego, which is that annoying nagging voice in our head, wants to keep us trapped in the past and/or worrying about the future. We will cover negative emotions in a while, but for now, just know that all negative emotions arise from not being present.

Again, if we observe small children, we will see that they are totally in the present moment and loving it all. I know most three year olds have few worries but we can learn a lot from them. The present moment is all we will ever have and it is the only place where we can create and progress our lives. Our lives are a series of now moments. The past and the future are merely illusions that our ego uses against us.

Our ego only wants to keep us "safe" and it has no interest in our happiness. If it can keep us focused on our past or future then it can distract us from making changes. Change equals danger to our ego so it does its best to distract us from the present moment. When we are present, we are either enjoying the moment or dealing with a situation. We are calm, relaxed and focused. There is no stress, worry or anger.

Whenever you are feeling bad, remember to ask yourself; "Am I present now?" This awareness will bring you back to the present.

Good versus bad

In our western world we think in terms of duality or opposites. We live in a world where we are very quick to judge events and people as good or bad. This leads to great fluctuations in our moods. We are encouraged to have strong opinions, one way or the other, as this is seen as a sign of conviction, decisiveness and intellect.

However, this labelling of everything as either good or bad can lead us onto the emotional rollercoaster of life. We tend to react strongly to events and people on first impressions. I believe that good and bad are intimately linked. They are part of a continuum and are not diametrically opposed to each other. You cannot have the concept of good without the concept of bad.

I will use an example that happened to me last week to illustrate the point. I was out in a restaurant with friends when I started to moan and complain about my steak being overdone. My first reaction was to label this event as bad. Then I realised that in order for me to judge this meal as bad; I must be lucky enough to have experienced plenty of good meals. This was a signal, that I noticed when I stopped complaining, that I am very blessed and fortunate. Imagine if we gave the same bad meal to a starving person. Would they complain like I had? No way. Their idea of a bad meal is no meal at all. Again it is a matter of changing our perspective and becoming more aware of our judgements.

Good and bad merge into one. We need to look at everything being part of the whole experience of life. If there was no bad then good could not exist. You would have no reference point for good if you had not experienced bad. If there was no cloud, there could not be a silver lining and vice versa. Just remember that the next time you feel unhappy, it just means that you must have known happiness. Be grateful for this realisation and for your past and future happiness. This means that everything that is bad in your life must have an element of good. There is a golden nugget in every situation. Just accept that sometimes the good does not reveal itself until days, months or even years later. Everything that happens, happens for the best. I am sure you have experienced this as well. This takes a little time to get your head around as you are trying to change a lifetime of thinking a certain way. It is like learning to eat with your weak hand; it can be done but it just takes time and practice. Time and repetitive practice are our friends here.

I used to get frustrated if things did not work out as I expected. Now I realise that everything that slows me down is there to help me. Everything that gets in my way is a gift in some way.

For every left, there must be a right. If we are down then there must be an up. To feel cold, you must have felt warm. You get the idea. If we can stop labelling everything in opposite terms of good and bad, we can view everything as just being. We need to stop listening to others as to how we should react to life and follow our own, more enlightened path.

Turn that off

If we realise that we are our thoughts, then we must learn to control and guard our minds. We must be careful who we listen to and also what we place into our minds. We need a constant supply of positive and healthy material to feed our minds with. Think of your mind as fertile soil; if you plant weeds then weeds will grow. If you plant flowers then they will grow and blossom.

One area that has a great effect on our lives is the media; newspapers, magazines, radio and television. We have to remember that these all exist in order to make money. They are businesses that survive by selling primarily advertising space. In order to charge top rate for adverts, they need as high an audience or readership as possible. These businesses will therefore feed us with any old garbage that the public wants. They have little interest in the truth but just give their consumers whatever they want. This is why five newspapers will have five different headings, as they are designed to satisfy their own readership.

Bad news sells. We are fed a constant diet of negativity twenty-four hours a day. It is a wonder that we have the courage to leave our homes. The other day I watched a sixty second news summary and counted six negative stories and only one positive one. Indeed they often put a humorous story at the end of a depressing news story. This is probably to prevent their viewers from killing themselves so they will tune in to more rubbish the next day. How can this constant tirade of negativity be good for our happiness? It cannot. Negativity by definition can only have a negative effect on us.

There is enough misery in the world without us wallowing in more of it. Television is another area we must be careful with. I have no issue with the programme makers as they are trying to run a business. We just have to show more awareness of what we consume and only watch stuff that serves us. Winston Churchill was the Home Secretary when television was first introduced in the UK. He was appalled by it and referred to it as "the idiot's lantern" due to the fact that he thought it would rot the nation's brains. Unfortunately, mostly he was right.

There is a TV show on at present called "Take me out." Apparently in this game show around twenty attractive, intelligent young women beg and plead to be taken out by one lucky guy. Now I am guessing that a lot of the audience consists of young, teenage girls. Imagine how this impacts their sense of self-worth and self-esteem. Again nobody questions this.

There have been psychological studies done on people who have watched soap operas every day for the last twenty to thirty years. These people now exhibit signs of what is referred to as Soap Opera Syndrome. In short their lives become soap operas. We become what we think about, so after decades of watching inane, negative, violent drivel, they find themselves living out some sordid soap opera in their lives. I am not judging here as this is just an observation. Just look at the breakdown in the fabric of families and society. These programmes are not entirely to blame, but any rational person can see they cannot help but drag us all down.

The movie industry is also far from blameless. You have probably seen the smash hit film "Titanic." Apart from being historically inaccurate and an insult to the families of many of the participants, it has a deep, underlying message. Throughout this film all the villains were rich and the heroes were all poor. In one scene the rich villain (Rose's husband) even had the poor people in third class locked in as the ship sunk. This never happened of course. In another scene the heroine, Rose, is having a dreary meal in the first class restaurant. In due course she escapes to the lower decks where all the poor people are having a fantastic time singing and dancing. The message is clear; it is terrible and evil to be rich and wonderful to be poor. Many novels and films carry this anti-wealth, anti-success message. Conclusion; be careful what you watch.

I try to watch, listen and read only positive content. This makes you into a bit of a weirdo as you cannot participate in endless, mindless conversations about the latest celebrity talent show. People will think you are even a little strange. What other people think is, however, their business and not ours. We are interested and focused on our happiness. We cannot change others, just ourselves. I keep away from soaps, news and politics, violence and all celebrity game shows. I do watch comedies, sport, nature, science and history programmes. I have little use for the rest.

When you are without, go within

Captain Jerry Coffee was a US Navy Pilot on active service in Vietnam. One day he was shot down and taken prisoner by the Viet Cong. They placed him in solitary confinement and chained him to the floor of his small cell. During seven years of captivity, Captain Coffee survived numerous beatings, a starvation diet, disease and stifling heat.

After his release he said that his survival was due to the fact that he learnt to mentally switch off from his hellish existence. He did this by using faith. Firstly he got strength by his faith in God. Secondly he drew great strength in his faith in himself to survive. He did this by exercising in his cell every day, and by visualising his past and mentally experiencing a brighter future. Thirdly he developed great faith in his fellow prisoners of war.

The prisoners developed a form of "tap code." They used this code to communicate support to each other. Jerry even learnt to speak French by tapping through the walls to another prisoner! Lastly Jerry kept the faith with his country. He realised that the propaganda, that the communists were feeding them each day, was designed to break their spirit. The prisoners kept their military discipline and structure, even though this was against the rules. Amazingly Jerry learnt the names of over six hundred prisoners. The reason was that, if he ever got released then he could inform the men's relatives that they were still alive. After seven long years Jerry was released. Today he is a world famous speaker who shares his unique story.

Perhaps we should all learn from Jerry. When life is seemingly hopeless we too need to keep the faith. When we are without we must go within and draw upon reserves of inspiration and strength that we never knew we had. It is not what is happening on the outside but rather what is going in on the inside that will determine our destiny. I just wanted to share this story with you as I found it so inspiring.

Negative emotions

We all have no problem with experiencing positive, happy emotions. We are entitled to them, indeed happiness is our natural state. However, due to a lifetime of negative input that we have discussed, our thinking tends to steer us towards a negative view of ourselves and the world. We have two choices; we can view the world as a mostly benevolent place or as being malevolent. The first choice lets us realise that the world is filled with mainly good people and experiences with a minority of bad. The latter choice gives us the opposite view.

Our own experiences are proof that we live in a benevolent world and an abundant universe. This is an empowering belief system and one that will help us in life. We need to observe our negative thoughts and ask ourselves "How is this thought helping me?" If it is not helping us then it is taking us further away from what we want to achieve. It is therefore of no use and needs to be discarded like any rubbish we generate. Put it in the rubbish bin marked negative emotions and get them buried in landfill. We do not want them recycled. Again this is a slow, gradual process of increasing our awareness of our thoughts and exercising greater control over them. It is not easy but it is certainly worth the prize; the prize of lasting contentment.

Buddha said "All we are is the result of what we have thought." Centuries later Earl Nightingale said "Your world is a living expression of how you are using and have used your mind." Both these quotes tell us how important our thoughts are, as they are the primary way in which we create our reality and life.

We need to spend some time then, analysing our negative thoughts and realising that: 1. They are of no use to us and 2. We can discard them and replace them with thoughts that better serve us. We must also remember that we can only hold one conscious thought at a time. That thought needs to be positive or we will fill that void with a negative. Nature hates a vacuum so we have to be proactive in our thinking and not reactive to daily events. We must not take chances with our own happiness.

Let us now explore the thoughts that can trap us into a spiral of negativity. These are in no particular order but we all suffer from them to varying degrees.

Worry

We live in a world of worry. This is hardly surprising when we are surrounded by negativity. This constant negative input heightens our worrying and anxiety. We watch the news and worry about interest rates rising, the economy, our job security and global warming. It is little wonder that our minds quickly become preoccupied by all this bad stuff. When we worry we are taken out of the present moment. Why? Because we worry about something which might happen in the future. This takes our focus off the present moment, which is the only place that we can create our future. Now there is a paradox.

We talked earlier about the importance of being present. When we are present we can focus on now. Instead of worrying, we can plan our future. This is a subtle and important difference. We can only really enjoy life when we are fully engaged in the present moment. Life is uncertain by its nature, which of course leads us to worry. The solution here is to draw strength from the fact that we have dealt with every tough situation life has thrown at us. The fact that you are reading this now is proof of that.

This should be a great source of strength to draw upon. Think of all the difficult times that you have dealt with. You probably have come out of them wiser and stronger. It states in the Bible that we should be grateful for our difficulties. They are sent to help us and let us grow. Think about Jerry Coffee; his hardships sculpted him into a world class person in every respect. You cannot create champions on a feather bed.

When we worry, are we focusing on what we want or what we don't want? This is negative goal setting. We are thinking about, and therefore giving energy to, what we hope does not happen. The law of attraction states that we attract into our lives what we think about. If we worry, not only do our worries seem to grow, but we attract even more worries. This is madness, but it does not stop us all from doing it.

A big cause of worry is <u>indecision.</u> I am at my worst when I cannot make a decision. Nothing is better for increasing anxiety and worry than being indecisive. The solution, therefore, is simple. Make more decisions. It is said that successful people make decisions quickly and are slow to change them. Most people, if they ever do make a decision, are quick to change it.

I find that if I have a problem that is worrying me, my best course of action is to: 1. Write out the problem. 2. List all possible solutions. 3. List the pros and cons of each solution and 4. Make a decision and write it down. If we put our problem on paper it creates a gap between us and the problem. Defining a problem also makes us look objectively at it. Often, especially in a state of worry, we increase the size of our problems beyond reality. Remember; winners think on paper.

When I have written down my solution, I suddenly feel much better. I can now focus on a constructive solution instead of wasting my time worrying. This frees me up to take action and to move forward. We have already said that happiness equals progress. Therefore being stuck in worry is the last place we want to find ourselves.

<u>Fear</u>

The next cancer of the mind we need to explore is fear. Fear is our mortal enemy. We fear our future, we fear for our health, our finances and failure itself. There are only two states that we find ourselves in; fear or faith. This book is about building faith in your unique abilities and talents. Fear is the worst destroyer of our dreams, as it can stop us from even trying.

Like our friend worry, fear is often nothing to do with any present danger to us. It is usually about what might happen in the future. As there are an infinite number of possibilities in the future, we would drive ourselves crazy if we thought of them all. FEAR is therefore about trying to deal with something that may not happen. Psychologists tell us that only 10% of our fears and worries actually happen.

You may well have heard that fear is an acronym for False Evidence Appearing Real. Again it is our perception of reality and what could happen that causes our fears. As the future does not exist then our fears are actually illusions. Just like in the film, we are trapped in our own matrix; the matrix of fear. This causes us to play it safe and not to dare to stretch ourselves.

The inventor James Dyson often says that you will never learn from your successes but only your failures. The founder of IBM, Tom Watson, once told a reporter that if you want to increase your success, then you must double your rate of failure. Why is it then, that we are all so scared of failure? Again I think social conditioning has a lot to do with it. Do you remember at school that if you got a sum wrong, then the teacher gave us a red X. You were effectively punished for making a mistake. This conditioned us to not experiment too much or raise our heads over the parapet. We quickly learnt not to take too many risks, as in school there is only one correct answer. In life, though, there are often many correct answers and multiple wrong ones.

Success lives on the far side of failure. Most successful people have endured multiple failures before they were a success. Also if you make a mistake and learn from it, you are closer to finding the right way. This is called progress. I can only wonder what James Dyson's friends thought when he gave up his city career to pursue his dream. He spent years taking apart old vacuum cleaners before he successfully invented "The Dyson."

The antidote for fear is preparation. The better prepared we are the less we have to fear. The emperor Napoleon was a master tactician. He analysed everything that could go wrong before a battle started. He then created a plan for every eventuality. Another way to minimise our fears is to ask the question; "What is the worst thing that could happen?" You will find that, in even the worst case scenario, there are benefits to be had.

Fear stops us from taking risks and truly living. Life is the ultimate high risk game, in that none of us are getting out of it alive. We might as well play this game and enjoy the risks that make our journey so interesting. We all need uncertainty and, as we live in an uncertain universe, we may as well embrace risk.

Theodore Roosevelt famously said that we have nothing to fear, but fear itself. We must prepare for the worst but always expect the best. All our fears are located between our own ears. When we look at the vastness of the universe, then our greatest fears truly are insignificant. In a million years from now they will be even less important. Let's keep our fears in perspective and realise that all our possessions will be left behind when we leave this world. Perhaps then it is time to take more risks. The worst thing fear does is to stop us from growing. Growth is at the very core of leading a happy, productive life.

Depression

This is the biggie. This ranges from sadness to low moods, and all the way to clinical depression. Nothing weakens our immune system, lowers our energy and destroys our resolve better than depression. Again the last gift in Pandora's Box was hope. When there is seemingly no hope, then depression can strike the strongest of us down. In the Bible it says "My people perish for lack of a vision." How true; we all need an empowering vision.

We must always keep in mind that our thought patterns are largely habitual. Therefore we have often got into the habits of feeling bad. As a carer, the physical and psychological pressures on us can often seem overwhelming. This is when we are at our most vulnerable. If our mind is like a garden, then we must be proactive and take out the weeds as they appear. We particularly need to dig out the old tough weeds whose roots have grown deep and strong.

It is inevitable that we will have bad days. When we do, the more tools we have to combat our bad feelings the better we are able to cope. The better the chances of recovering quickly from our low mood. Depression saps our physical resources which leads to physical illness. Our thoughts can make us sick so we owe it to ourselves to fight this malaise.

Our first place to focus is of course our physiology. It is really a process of observation and awareness. A stitch in time saves nine. The earlier we can self-diagnose that we are feeling bad, the quicker we can rectify it and therefore suffer less. Change your body as quickly as you can by movement, breathing and by using your vision. Recapture your energy.

Medical research definitely points to a lack of sleep as being a factor in a lot of low level depression. One hour before midnight is better than two after, as my old granny used to say. It turns out she was right. There are certain chemicals that our brain needs that it can only produce when we are asleep.

Eating a healthy diet and avoiding processed, junk food is also key. Fresh vegetables, fruit and grains contain a lot of vitamins and minerals that keep both body and mind healthy. We need to always remember that the two are linked and indeed are really the same.

Next we must constantly feed our minds with good, positive material. The heroes in this book show us that it is possible to grow in the most challenging situations. If we don't keep the good stuff coming in then the bad stuff will get us. There is more than enough bad stuff in the world to keep us depressed for ten lifetimes. We are all susceptible to this rubbish so let's keep guard on our mind. It is the little things in life that make the big difference. We just need to focus on feeling good. Keep your mind on your goals and the things you want. Read your list of the things that make you happy and just do one of them. It all makes a difference.

I believe that our happiness in life is proportionate to our gratitude. The more grateful we are the happier we are. Focus on increasing your gratitude list each day. I know these things take time. You are not wasting your time here, you are investing it. You are ensuring your health and creating energy. With this energy you can better help yourself and others. Your attitude will positively affect others. You will be more productive. You will live longer. This is a big claim but success is often a few simple disciplines practiced every day.

When I am feeling down you can probably guess who I am thinking about. Myself of course. We have a natural tendency to mentally go within ourselves and withdraw from the world. This is my danger signal that I am about to have an acute attack of PLOM disease. I heard the speaker Zig Ziglar use this phrase. It stands for Poor Little Old Me. I have a one man pity party where nobody comes or brings me presents. If I catch myself doing this then my solution is to get my mind off me and onto someone else. It's time to phone a friend as they say. One of the great things about caring for another person is that your focus is off yourself. People who serve others are often the happiest people in our society. I am sure your life experiences have proved this to be true.

Sadness is often a signal that one of our human needs is, temporarily at least, in deficit. We all have a need for love and connection. I will stick my neck out here and say that women are more prone to depression than men. I believe that women have a higher need for love and connection than men. They need it at a deeper level. It is central to their core and well-being. A lot of women experience great pain when their children leave home, for example. That incredibly strong bond a woman has with her children feels broken. Women also need to connect with their partners on a deeper level that often baffles us men! We cannot always change our circumstances but, at least if we can identify what we are needing, we can take some action. We have all felt bad but have not known why. Self-knowledge is key here. We need to be our best friend, coach and cheer leader. We must understand and love ourselves unconditionally.

Anger

This is possibly the most dangerous emotion and certainly the most destructive to our health. Anger causes huge problems in our society. Many people are languishing in prison because they could not control their anger. Often anger is again an impulsive reaction to a situation that we judge as negative.

We often feel anger when we are frustrated. I still feel this anger welling up whenever I have a computer problem. The key as always is awareness of our changing emotions. I remind myself again that the things that slow us down are sent to help us. I try to remember this when things frustrate me. This frustration is a sign that I need to learn a lesson instead of boiling over with anger. Our negative emotions can be good if we can quickly learn the lesson and be grateful for this new insight. If we can feel good about our negative emotions then we instantly change them into a positive.

What gender do you think spends the most time in anger management classes? You guessed it; men. Again this is often down to the testosterone flying around men's bloodstreams. A certain level of aggression is needed to be effective in sports and life. There is a positive side to everything and men, in particular, must focus on channelling our aggression into positive areas such as exercise. If we return again to the six human needs, what the problem here is often our need for significance.

Society and genetics have given men a very high need for significance. Men often feel anger when this need is not met i.e. by losing face. I used to feel anger if I thought anyone was being rude or disrespectful. This of course was getting in the way of my need for respect or significance. Now that I realise what is going on this helps to lessen the feelings. Diagnosis is half the cure as they say.

A great danger with anger is the damage we do to ourselves. Buddha said that being angry with someone is like throwing a red hot rock at them. You may hurt them but you will definitely hurt yourself! The Chinese have a saying that the man who seeks revenge must dig two graves. Whenever someone tries to hurt you then remember they have already lost. They are certainly hurting themselves with their anger. Just allow them to blow themselves out (anger is very tiring). You do not have to like what they are saying. I tend to avoid these unpleasant exchanges by not fighting back. I tend to just smile. I will not let myself get into a harmful argument. No one wins an argument anyway. Just tell the person you will talk to them when they calm down. They will soon get the message.

We human beings are nothing more than sophisticated Chimpanzees. Like most animals, especially mammals, we live in a strictly hierarchical system. Status is everything. If we lose status, especially males, then we lose respect and our position in society. This is probably why so many men die within a couple of years of retirement. They lose their status and often their purpose.

Anger stops the natural flow of energy in our bodies. Just ask yourself how you feel when you are angry. Not good I bet. Angry people live short, tormented lives. Our job is not to be one of them.

Regret

Who does not have any regrets? The lesson here to learn is simple: if you are having regrets then you are not present. We only regret the past. If we are trapped in the past then we cannot create in the present moment. The past is past and what can we do about it? Nothing, so there is no place for regret. If we fully accept where we are right now then there can be no regrets.

The past does not exist and is therefore an illusion. If you do not believe me then try showing someone your past.

You can only show someone the effects of the past. The past only existed when it was the present. You may need to read that again to let that sink in. When I understood this my whole life changed. I had spent a considerable amount of time and effort thinking and regretting past mistakes and decisions. I would waste my time thinking about something that no longer exists, that I cannot change and only makes me feel bad. If you think about it, this is total madness!

You have probably said something like: "If I had my time again I would do …" Yes, of course we all think this but is it useful to us? Life is not a dress rehearsal. We cannot edit our lives later. It is a live show. This is probably why things go wrong. We can only try to grab life's lessons as they happen and adapt our thinking and actions as we go along. A useful phrase here is to say to yourself often the following: "I will figure it out as I go along." The things we regret often turn out to be the best thing that could have happened anyway.

We need to realise that everything happens for a reason. The past is gone forever and all we have is the present moment. Again I would recommend "The Power of Now" by Eckhart Tolle which explains the idea of being present and its importance to our happiness.

Resentment

You cannot resent what you want. This is such an important statement and one we need to really understand. Resentment is another emotion and thought pattern that holds no value for us. Here is a good saying: "Bless what you want." In other words we must not resent someone who has what we want.

A lot of people resent wealthy people. Secretly they yearn for wealth and millions play the lottery. The problem is that you are resenting what you secretly desire. Can you see how confusing this is for your subconscious? If you won the lottery you would have to resent yourself! Often we give ourselves mixed messages and this is why we get mixed results. Did you know that the vast majority of lottery winners end up poorer within five years of their big win? Whatever we desire, we have to emotionally connect to it. We have to celebrate the success of others. If we resent someone then we just end up attracting more resentment into our lives. This takes us away from our desires.

The next time you see someone who has a great body, relationship, money, etc. silently bless them. You can even go up to them and say "Wow you look great, what's your secret?" The great thing is that they will often tell you. This is a win-win as they feel better, you feel good and you have just learnt something in the process. It just goes against the grain of a lifetime's conditioning.

Judgement

Another habit we must drop is judgement. This is something we have been taught by society to do. It is another bad habit which we have picked up and never questioned. It is seen as a type of strength by many people. I believe it shows weakness of character. If I judge someone to be lazy, stupid, rude or even all three then how does this help me? If I am judging someone negatively then I am thinking negatively. We know that there is no place in our life for negativity. Even if we are accurate in our assessment, the fact we are right does not help us.

Judgement is weakness because often we judge because we are too lazy to get the facts. Judgement is easy. It does not require much thought if any. Judgement leads us to label people. We are all more than just a label. If we had all the facts then we may not need to label someone at all. Again we must observe without judgement.

People who are highly judgemental are often hiding their own low self-esteem. By judging we are often justifying to ourselves that we are somehow superior to them. If we have a healthy, positive self-esteem then we do not need to compare ourselves to others. We have no need for boasting, criticism and judgement as they reinforce our insecurities. I hope you are now convinced that judgement really is weakness. This is a weakness we can do without.

Guilt

I remember the day that my mum went into a home. Along with the sense of relief that she was in the best place to receive the care she needed, a strong sense of guilt rose up in me. This sense of guilt haunted me for many weeks. Could I have done more to keep her in her own place? Will the loss of her independence finish her? Why am I out with friends enjoying myself? After giving this matter much thought I found a better meaning. The reason I was feeling guilty was because I cared. This was a revelation and comfort to me.

I had done my best, like most people do, and now her condition had made it necessary for my mum to receive a higher level of professional care. I had not always been perfect but God did not make me perfect. I had found acceptance. I had to accept what had happened and move on. I am glad to say that the home made my mum's final few years comfortable ones.

Guilt is another life sapping thought pattern. Everyone does the best they can in any given situation, so what is there to feel guilty about? Yes, we have all done things that we regret and would do differently. Acceptance again is the key here. We must accept our mistakes, learn from them and move on. We cannot change the past, only our future by focusing on the present moment.

Guilt is often used by other people against us. "If you cared about me you would….." We must not let guilt manipulate us. We do things because they feel right to us and are in line with our values. People will soon realise that you are not catching their guilt and give up. Guilt cannot serve us as it makes us feel bad. We know that feeling bad cannot make us happy. We have been brought up to feel guilty so we think it is normal. It should not be normal to feel bad.

Be responsible

By now you should be excited at all the tools you have at your disposal. It is our responsibility to use them to ensure our ongoing contentment. Remember that the things that are easy to do are also easy not to do. We must discipline ourselves to use these skills in our daily lives.

Pretty soon someone is going to rain on your parade. People who are negative love to spread it around. We cannot always control how other people talk and act. We can only focus on how we respond to these events. Even in a heated argument we must keep a little back and try to observe ourselves. This act of observance increases our awareness that we are being dragged down the route of negativity.

Don't become a victim

We have discovered earlier that we never experience reality but merely our perception of reality. We also know that there is no good or bad as such. Eleanor Roosevelt once said "No one can make you feel inferior without your permission." For years I tacitly gave people the right to make me feel bad. As soon as I allowed this then the other person was controlling my thoughts and emotions. I needed to get away from the idea that "You are making me angry." If I changed it to "I am allowing you to make me angry" then I was accepting responsibility for my emotions.

This new way of thinking stated that, from now on I was 100% responsible for my thoughts. I could no longer play the victim. Everything I think, good or bad, is my fault. We are all the captain of our own ship. Often we will be battered off course by the inevitable storms of life. We must constantly make small and sometimes large corrections. We must keep our eyes on the prize until we get there. There is great power in the word until. How long will we persist in our search for life's treasures? Until we get there.

Conclusion

If we are what we think then let's make our thoughts better. The great news is that there is no limit to how well we can think. The better we think then the better our lives will become.

We cannot always change our lives but we are all powerful as to how we think. We have seen through the story of Jerry Coffee that it is possible to reframe any experience. We can grow through adversity and turn negatives into priceless treasures. The only place that negativity exists is between our ears. It is time to kill off this life destroying bug. We have the power to do this. It is our duty and natural state to be happy.

What we need to do is fan the flames of desire. Imagine the power you would have if you had total control over your mind. You would be indestructible. Imagine what you could do for others. The highest prize in life is peace of mind. It is achievable if we practice daily to improve our thinking.

There is no inherent meaning in any given event. We give events meaning through our thinking. If we improve our thinking then we change the meaning we give to life's ups and downs. This is exactly why people can grow in the most challenging of conditions. They have found a better, more empowering meaning. This meaning has given them hope, energy and a new purpose. This is something that we all can do. It is our natural destiny to grow. Trying to create the life we want with negative emotions is like trying to drive with the hand brake on. It is time to release our negative emotions which are the brakes to our success.

Action points

- Resolve to be happy now. Feeling good attracts more good things into our lives. Do not put your happiness off for a future event that may never happen.
- Avoid measuring yourself in terms of your material possessions. Never compare yourself to others. Compare yourself to your goals. Progress is everything.

- Stay focused on what you want.
- Practice calming your mind often. Bring in no mind at least once a day. Prove to yourself that you are in control of your thoughts.
- Avoid negative situations, people, TV, Films and reading materials. Keep feeding yourself with the positive and you will keep out the negative.
- Accept what is. You will be much happier.
- Stay in the present moment. Another word for the present is a gift. Appreciate and use this gift.
- Analyse your negative emotions as they surface. What is this telling me? What do I need here? Always look for a positive meaning. This way you can always turn bad into good. You have the power.

CONCLUSION

"You make a living by what you get. You make a life by what you give." – Sir Winston Churchill

I believe the greatest gift you can give anyone is your own personal development. I say this because, for a lot of people, spending time improving yourself can be viewed as being selfish. Nothing could be further from the truth. If we are happier, stronger, more resilient, wiser and healthier then we are in a much better position to help others. People will enjoy being around you and your positivity will rub off on them. How can this be selfish?

George Bernard Shaw once said: "This is the ***true joy in life***, the being used for a purpose recognized by yourself as a mighty one; the being thoroughly worn out before you are thrown on the scrap heap; the being a force of Nature instead of a feverish selfish little clod of ailments and grievances complaining that the world will not devote itself to making you happy." It is easy to retreat into our shells when life is tough. What you are doing, by reading this book, is to attempt the opposite. This takes guts. Congratulate yourself for this; you deserve your brighter future.

What you are doing is really investing in yourself. Few people do this because they would rather just complain.

Change is not easy but it can be fun. It is a fascinating journey. Any journey is better than standing still. It is my profound wish that the information in this book will make your journey more enjoyable for yourself and those closest to you. Above all, this book should leave you with practical actions that you can fit in around your schedule. Please do not get overwhelmed and just do what feels right for you.

Success is often just doing small daily disciplines on a consistent basis. These small disciplines, like going for a thirty minute walk each day or reading, slowly build up and will make a huge difference. Albert Einstein said that compounding was the eighth wonder of the world. We will never know what the smallest action will do to our future. These small acts compound over time and give us the feeling of progress. And we already know that happiness equals progress.

Educational physiologists tell us that we are lucky to retain 30% of what we read. In a few short weeks you will have forgotten most of this book. Any book that is worth reading once is worth reading again. Make your education a daily habit as you do with washing. Think of your reading as daily maintenance or the cleansing of your mind. Nothing is more important or more enjoyable than getting to know yourself. The more you like yourself, of course, the more you will like others. People will notice these changes in you before you will. They will notice that you carry yourself better, that you are happier and more optimistic. You will look and feel younger. These are bold claims but you are just using all the universal laws in your favour. You are swimming with the tide. You are no longer struggling but are allowing the good things into your life. You are becoming an unstoppable force for good as you gain momentum. Yes, life will still throw its nasty surprises at you. The difference now is that you will find that little nugget of golden wisdom in every setback and mistake. What does not kill us makes us stronger. Everything always happens for a reason whether it is seemingly good or bad.

Now I want to recap the seven chapters of this book. Repetition is the mother of learning. It is the master skill for us all to use in order to develop our understanding.

CHAPTER ONE – MENTORS

In this first chapter we discussed the importance of finding great mentors or role models. Often we try to struggle and reinvent the wheel. This is often because it is seen as a sign of weakness to ask for help. This is not helpful thinking. Why not tap into the wisdom and experiences of others?

The great news is that mentors are all around us. We just have to find and identify them. People like to help others. Allow someone the opportunity to help you and feel better as a result. If you think about it that way you are both gaining. I have heard it said that teaching is the highest form of learning. I have certainly learnt a great deal by writing this book. I can thank you for that. If we can think win-win in every interaction we have we will improve ourselves and the lives of everyone we meet.

We all have barriers to overcome. Mine was shyness. I had to realise that I was letting my shyness master me. It was holding me back. It was not allowing me to contribute fully. Once I had identified the problem I could deal with it. Whatever we want in life someone else has in abundance.

Start looking for your dream team. You can find inspiration from the people around you, at work, in books and on the internet. I have found that reading the stories of people who have overcome huge challenges particularly inspiring. I like to study ordinary people who have done extraordinary things. We need to be grateful for and appreciate their achievements. They have left a trail for us to follow. Gratitude and appreciation for others are purely positive thoughts. They will help us attract the people, knowledge and resources that we need. Let's all learn from the experts. This is the quickest route to our desires.

CHAPTER TWO – INTEGRITY

One day a little boy was playing at home when his dad arrived home after a long day at work. The father still had a lot of work to do but that did not stop his son from pestering his dad to play with him. The father noticed a magazine on the table with a picture of a map of the world on it. He quickly cut the picture into many pieces and told his son to come back when he had taped the picture back together. He figured that he would get at least half an hour of peace that way.

A few minutes later the boy gave the completed map back to his dad. Surprised by this, the dad asked him how he had done this so quickly. The little boy smiled and said; "I just turned the pieces over and there was a picture of a man. All I did was put the man together and then the world came together."

This chapter is about putting ourselves together. The word integrity means wholeness. We are putting our mind, body and spirit together. We are re-engineering ourselves like a golfer would with his swing.

Integrity of the mind starts with our values. This is why I asked you to write out your top ten values. These are what your life is about. You already know this stuff but the act of writing them down, clarifies them. This list can change as your life changes but the core values will always remain. They are your foundation. The stronger the foundation the higher the building can reach. You will also be better able to resist the negative influences of the outside world. Your values will not shift with popular opinion, or by what is perceived by society as politically correct or trendy. Nothing and no one can take your values from you. They are your treasures to keep.

We discussed that a healthy body creates a healthy mind. Good health is everything and is central to a great life. Most health problems today arise from our lifestyles. We all enjoy a better standard of living than previous generations and have access to far superior medical services. On top of this the internet is a great source of medical and health information. In spite of all these advances, problems such as obesity and heart conditions have risen dramatically in recent decades.

The answer here is simple. Live like our grandparents did. They ate little to no processed foods, drank less and got more sleep and exercise. One of the best things you can do for your future is to resolve to increase your general health and fitness. As with everything else just start where you can. It is advisable to get medical advice and a full check up to see where you are physically. This can be daunting, especially for us men, but we need to start with the truth. Make continuous small adjustments to your diet.

Get into an exercise or sport that will not hurt you and you will enjoy. Build up slowly but surely. With weight loss it is easy to measure your progress. What gets measured improves. Remember to do the simple things, such as parking furthest away and taking the stairs instead of the lift. It all adds up. Never underestimate the power of walking. The human body was designed for movement. Gradually you will feel stronger and healthier. You cannot buy this feeling and you will not want to go back to a sedentary lifestyle.

If you just cut sugar out of your diet, you will notice a huge difference. You will lose weight and feel younger. We know that sugar and salt are in all processed foods. We are not trying to be perfect, we are just cutting back. We must still treat ourselves now and then. Be sure to eat up your greens. We discussed the great health benefits of alkaline foods, so refer to the list I gave you earlier.

You cannot drink enough water. As we are 80% water this is what our body craves the most. Most people are dehydrated. This is not good. Drink water constantly during the day. You will have more energy and your skin will look better. Your body needs water to burn calories and to flush out all those toxins we ingest. We also said that rest is essential to a long, healthy life. Turn the TV and internet off and go to bed earlier. You will feel happier and will function better. We do not pay the price for good health; we enjoy the benefits.

Thirdly we talked about the spiritual side of ourselves. I laid out what I believed. I believe that there is a part of everyone that is spiritually perfect. If you are a believer then I encourage you to practice your religion or spirituality. This feeling of oneness with something greater than us puts our lives in perspective. It will strengthen your physical and mental health. You will find the inner peace and calm that is in us all.

CHAPTER THREE – NEW

When was the last time you did something for the first time? This is such a great question to ask ourselves, so I thought I would repeat it. It is easy for life to become a repetitive routine. This can lead to boredom, dissatisfaction and ultimately depression. The antidote to this is to incorporate and utilise the power of bringing the new into our lives.

We talked about how human beings need uncertainty in their life. This is why sport is so addictive. It is the uncertainty of the result that keeps us glued to the screen. It is the same with our lives. We need a level of uncertainty. The best way to bring this in is to try something new. It could be a new hobby, a new habit, a new career or a new country to visit. The more variety we can bring into our lives the better. We are all in the habit of waiting. We are all going to start something tomorrow. Why not start now? We need to break the habit of our routine where we can. We all deserve a little excitement.

We mentioned the importance of developing new skills. It does not have to be serious so why not learn to juggle, dance or use the computer. Hobbies are a great way of losing yourself in a passion. This renews your energy and zest for life. This will help you to better care for your loved ones. We all need a break from time to time. Even those with the tightest resources can find a way. We can be creative in how we find the time and money to indulge ourselves.

How is your luck? Luck is a skill that we can acquire. If we follow the ideas covered in this chapter, we can greatly increase our luck. Who doesn't need that? Follow the strategies of lucky people and who knows what might happen.

Life is for living. We owe it to ourselves to bring a certain level of variety and excitement into our lives.

CHAPTER FOUR – DREAM

Focus on what you want. This is great advice and something we must remind ourselves to do as often as possible. In reality though, we tend to focus on what we do not want. This attracts more of what we do not want into our lives. On top of this we get the extra benefits of worry, anxiety, stress, depression, ill health and insomnia. It sounds crazy but it does not stop us from doing it.

The solution, again, is of course to focus solely on what you do want. We do this through goal-setting. This is where we decide what we want, write it down and take action to achieve it. This sounds too simple but let's not be fooled by its simplicity. We went through the goal-setting process in the chapter. Remember to set goals in the areas that are important to you. Use your values list as guidance here.

Refer to your goals often and visualise them coming true. You are shaping and creating your future by doing this. You are focused. Remember to pick out one goal as your definite major purpose in life. This will often involve helping others in some way. This could be something that you are already doing or something new. By writing down your goals you are putting yourself in the top 3% of society. Allow yourself to feel good about that.

Do not worry about failing to reach your goals. The act of setting goals greatly increases your chances of success. If you do not achieve your goals then perhaps it was not meant to be. Perhaps life has something even better in store for you. Failure does not frighten you anymore because you will always find the valuable lesson. Have fun with your goals. Allow yourself to be that small child at Christmas. The world would be a better place if everyone set goals. Remember too that it is not what you get in life that is valuable; it is what you become. Imagine the person you will become if you act on your goals. This is your gift to yourself and the world.

CHAPTER FIVE – STATE

In this chapter we discussed the importance of our state. We defined state as being our psychological, emotional and physical condition at any given moment. We discovered that it is what is going on inside of us that is important. Often we allow the events of our life to dictate our feelings and actions.

I believe that we can take back control of our state and with it our destiny. We often cannot control what happens to us. We must focus on what we can control. We must be proactive in making sure we control our state whatever life throws at us. We must not react angrily to life's disappointments. This is not easy but it can be achieved with a little knowledge and effort.

Our minds act as a filter system. They filter out information by deleting, distorting and generalising. We covered the science of this in some depth. What all this means is that we do not experience reality. We only experience our own unique version of it. Therefore nothing is 100% real. Everything that we have ever cried over, got angry over, worried or got depressed over, did not really happen. That should change how you view life.

It is always the story we tell ourselves that determines an events meaning. We have seen, through several stories, that successful people manage to find an empowering meaning in any given situation. This is how they grow through adversity. They turn negatives into positives. Let's use these people to inspire us to find a better meaning in all our problems. Again there is no inherent meaning in any situation; only the meaning we give it. This is the message here.

Use your physiology to keep in a good state. Keep your eyes in peripheral vision, keep an upright stance and walk with purpose. Breathe deeply and smile at everyone you meet. As you walk use affirmations discussed earlier such as "I like myself." Write out your list of things that make yourself feel good. Use the visualisation techniques when you get a chance. They are quick and easy. Remember to ask yourself better questions. Ask "what is great about this situation?" rather than "why does this always happen to me?" The right questions allow us to learn and to grow from every situation.

All these little things add up. It all matters. Anything that can keep us in a positive state is valuable. It is about increasing our awareness of what is going on inside us. The less time we spend in a negative state, the more we will enjoy our lives. Just realise that you now have the power. You are in control. We can change our states in an instant. Never doubt that this is possible for you.

CHAPTER SIX – EDUCATE

Never has it been more important to learn. We must all rediscover the joy of learning. This is another area that we associate with hard work. We need to think of learning as fun. This is an adventure. If you read a book you do not know where it will take you.

Children, before the school system knocks it out of them, have a natural desire to learn. They are curious. They want to get into everything. Their favourite words are how and why. We all need to get in touch with our inner child. People who constantly learn are healthier, mentally sharper and live longer. We all need to regularly work out our minds. Luckily there has never been so much information available to the average person. It is time we all took advantage of the information age. Learning gives us new insights and perspectives. It keeps us young.

We discussed that, if you read just thirty minutes a day, you would have read hundreds of books in just a few years. You would be constantly updating your knowledge and skills. Your confidence would grow. You will feel great about yourself. You would have invested your time wisely.

If you hate reading then there are alternative ways to learn. I often go on to YouTube and watch recordings of great speakers. My favourite speakers are Jim Rohn, Brian Tracy, Tony Robbins and Wayne Dyer. There are many others. This is like going to a free seminar. It is a constant source of ideas and inspiration. Give it a go. Audio recordings are another great way to learn. Turn your car into a mobile university. This is a good way to turn wasted time, such as commuting, into learning time. Again this is about creating a new habit. It is about exposing our minds to good, positive material. If we put in the positive we lessen the amount of negative, harmful stuff.

Set yourself the goal of learning. It could be a new skill that gives you a new direction. Learning is a lifelong process so don't rush. Just do a little but do it often. You will soon be hooked.

CHAPTER SEVEN – THINK

We become what we think about. If we want to become happy, optimistic, healthy and wise; we must control our thinking accordingly. Everything that we have in our lives, and everything we will ever have, is the result of how we think. If we increase the quality of our thoughts, then we increase the quality of our life.

To improve our thoughts we must first resolve to be happy. We cannot put this off to a future point. This is too risky. If you are happy now then you will attract more happiness. The reverse is true also. In order to be happy we must realise that all negative thinking is unnatural. We have learned to indulge in this by a society that regards negativity as normal. By their very nature fear, worry, guilt, resentment and anger all take us away from happiness. Therefore they are of no use to us. They take us in the opposite direction to where we want to go.

The next time you have a strong negative feeling, just relax. Ask yourself; "How is this thought helping me?" It is not. Therefore you do not need it. Throw it away. It is trash. Just accept that the bad thoughts will come. We were not designed to be perfect. Now you know that, with practice you can deal with them before they overwhelm you. Take your time here as we have to change the bad habits of a lifetime.

Remember that you cannot experience negativity in the present moment. You can only be depressed, angry or worried if you are thinking about the past or what might happen in the future. Ask yourself often; "Am I present now?" This will bring you back to the present moment. You can only create the life you want when you are present.

Avoid negative people, TV, books, films and other materials. Instead fill the void with anything positive.

There are no prizes in life for being negative. There is only more negativity. Negative people lead negative lives. If you slowly but surely cut out the negative influences from your life, you will feel much happier. Lastly, practice bringing in no mind whenever you can. This proves to yourself that you are gaining greater control over your mind. And, as I have said countless times in this book, happiness equal progress.

Existential Pain

As we have mostly concentrated on happiness in this book, we need to cover the following insight. The fact that we are alive means that we will experience a certain level of physical and emotional pain. This is the pain of existence. Remember that the only people who feel no pain are dead. We have to accept certain painful truths such as –

- We will get sick and one day we will die.
- Our loved ones will get sick and will also die one day.
- We have the power of choice.
- We will constantly feel some pain throughout our lives.

We must accept these facts. They are part of the deal. Some of us will experience more pain than others. Life is not fair. All we can do is play the hand that fate has dealt us. Again just accept what is. Concentrate on what you can control. Concentrate on thinking the best thoughts you can. Always reach for the best thought. The fact that we have the power to choose means that we will make mistakes. This will lead to pain. The pain of regret. Also we will never know what would have been if we did not make that choice to marry a certain person or take that job. Learn to appreciate this pain of life. It means you are alive.

The Dash

The other day I visited my mum and dad's grave. I must admit that I tend to avoid graveyards. It was a sunny spring day, however, so everything looks a little more cheerful in the sunshine. As I looked at the various head stones I had a realisation. Often we look at the dates of someone's life such as; 16th August 1927 – 23rd September 2011. Then it occurred to me that what we remember about someone is the dash between those dates. That little dash represent someone's life. In my parents' case it represents two lives well lived.

If you are reading this then you are in your own dash. Let's make our dash the best it can be.

Sharpen the saw

The Japanese have a word called Kaizen. It means to constantly improve. It is an entire philosophy of living, as well as a word. This idea enabled Japan to recover from abject defeat in the war to become a major super power in just a few decades. Tony Robbins has the following idea; CANI. It stands for Constant And Never ending Improvement. Stephen S. Covey wrote an international best-selling book called "The Seven Habits of Highly Effective People." He called his seventh habit "sharpen the saw." The saw represents our life.

All three ideas have the same message for us. We must constantly improve and refine our thinking, habits and actions. This gets us onto an upward spiral where we develop new insights, awareness and greater understanding. We become stronger and more resilient. The seven areas this book recommends you work on are —

1. Seek out and select great mentors.
2. Work on your integrity of mind, body and spirit.
3. Be proactive in trying new skills, habits and strategies.
4. Set your goals and focus on them.
5. Get into a great state and stay there.
6. Constantly learn and grow.
7. Think positive thoughts.

We are talking about change. Change happens slowly. Just focus on these seven areas and know you are on the right path. You cannot fail if you just keep going. Lao-Tzu said: "A journey of a thousand miles begins with a single step." Just keep putting one foot in front of the other. Momentum will slowly build. Try focussing on one area at a time. Read this book again and you will gain greater insights. I hope this book has inspired you to read others. Everything you do that adds to your happiness adds to the well-being of others. You owe this to yourself and everyone in your world.

We have come a long way together. They say that the teacher always receives the greatest lesson. I want to again thank you for giving me this opportunity to grow and learn. I am no expert on personal development. I just have a passion for leading a happy, purposeful and productive life. I am sure you do also and I hope this book helps.

Before I leave you I want to reproduce a speech made by President John Kennedy. This speech says a great deal about what we humans can achieve. It is about achieving the impossible...

"We choose to go to the moon. We choose to go to the moon in this decade and do the other things, not because they are easy, but because they are hard, because that goal will serve to organize and measure the best of our energies and skills, because that challenge is one that we are willing to accept, one we are unwilling to postpone, and one which we intend to win, and the others, too.

To be sure, all this costs us all a good deal of money... Space expenditures will soon rise some more ... for we have given this program a high national priority—even though I realize that this is in some measure an act of faith and vision, for we do not now know what benefits await us.

But if I were to say, my fellow citizens, that we shall send to the moon, 240,000 miles away from the control station in Houston, a giant rocket more than 300 feet tall, the length of this football field, made of new metal alloys, some of which have not yet been invented, capable of standing heat and stresses several times more than have ever been experienced, fitted together with a precision better than the finest watch, carrying all the equipment needed for propulsion, guidance, control, communications, food and survival, on an untried mission, to an unknown celestial body, and then return it safely to earth, re-entering the atmosphere at speeds of over 25,000 miles per hour, causing heat about half that of the temperature of the sun—almost as hot as it is here today—and do all this, and do it right, and do it first before this decade is out—then we must be bold.

Many years ago the great British explorer George Mallory, who was to die on Mount Everest, was asked why he wanted to climb it. He simply relied, "Because it is there."

"Well, space is there, and we're going to climb it, and the moon and the planets are there, and new hopes for knowledge and peace are there. And, therefore, as we set sail we ask God's blessing on the most hazardous and dangerous and greatest adventure on which man has ever embarked."

—President John F. Kennedy, September 12, 1962

The British Prime Minister, Benjamin Disraeli, once said the following words. "Most people die with their music still locked up inside them. I am so grateful to have been able to get 'my music' out to you in the form of this book."

I hope this book has inspired you to take what steps you can to improve your life and your future.

I look forward to your success,

Take care,

William Long
Summer 2014

SUGGESTED READING

I have listed below ten of the books that have helped and inspired me over the years. These are good places to start. I find books a great source of strength and I refer to them often. Enjoy your reading.

Awaken the Giant within – Tony Robbins

7 Strategies for Wealth and Happiness – Jim Rohn

Think and Grow Rich – Napoleon Hill

The Power of Self-Confidence – Brian Tracy

Change your Thoughts Change your Life – Dr Wayne Dyer

Creating a Bug Free Mind – Andy Shaw

The Art of Happiness – The Dalai Lama

The Millionaire Mind – T. Harv. Ecker s

Man's Search for Meaning – Victor Frankl

Turning Point – Dr Rohan Weerasinghe